PROTEIN SPARING MODIFIED FAST COOKBOOK

Maria and Craig Emmerich

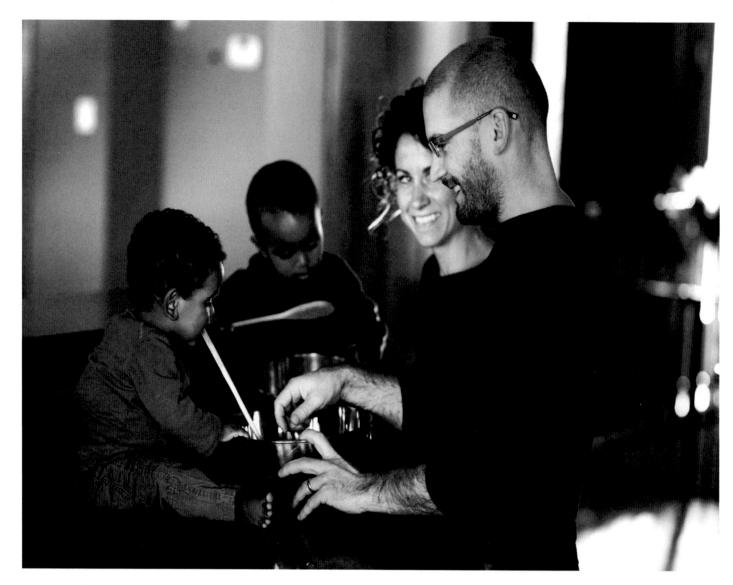

Thank You

I, like many of you, have had some really difficult times in my life. Life, like waves of the ocean, has high points as well as low points. It is during those low points that I had to stop spending money at restaurants and start cooking at home which helped me form into the healthy ketogenic cook I am today. I have learned to accept the low parts of the wave and to have gratitude for the high waves. The hardships taught me amazing life-long lessons. I struggled out of the cocoon and it made me a butterfly with strong wings.

I am grateful to my love and best friend, Craig, who never complains even though I often mess up the kitchen as soon as he cleans it. He has also been a huge part of this book: picking up all the groceries, testing recipes, as well as adding the detailed nutritional information for all the recipes.

I am grateful for my boys Micah and Kai who love to help me in the kitchen. Even though it takes twice as long to get dinner on the table when they help me, it is totally worth it. When we had to put our adoption on hold I was completely devastated, but I remember my mom telling me that my children just weren't born yet... I cry as I write this because she was totally right. These two boys were meant for me!

I want to express my gratitude to you, the reader! I can't thank you enough for all your love and support through my journey!

Contents

CONDIMENTS

SNACKS

SWEET TREATS

MEAL PLANS

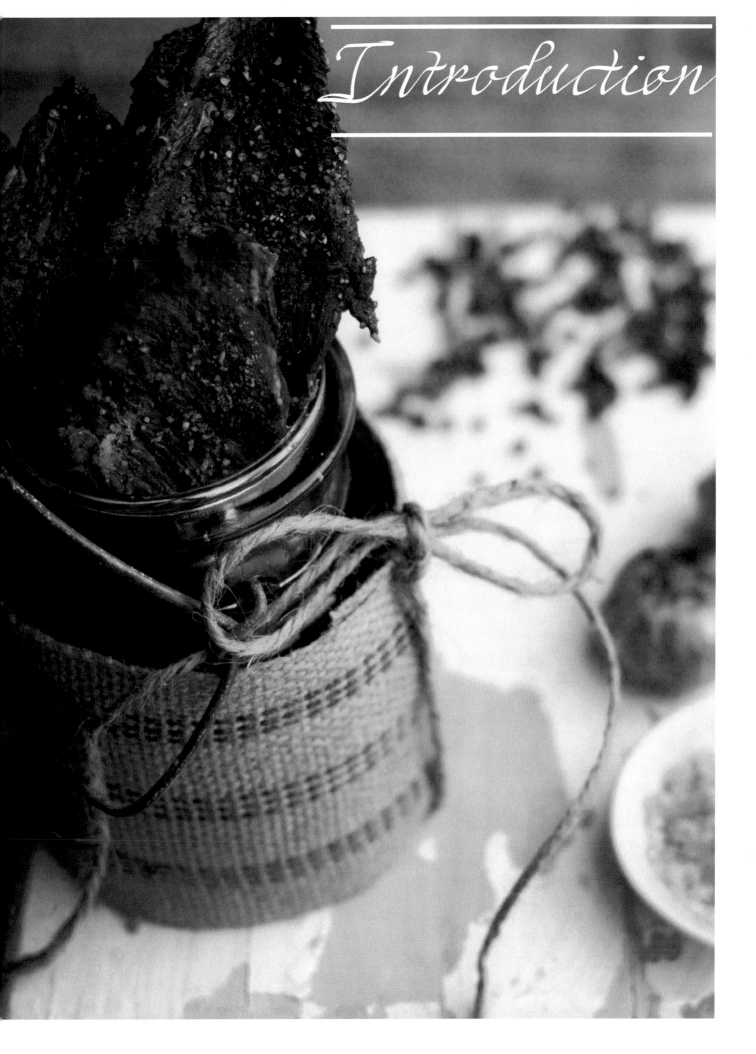

WHAT IS A PROTEIN SPARING MODIFIED FAST?

Protein Sparing Modified Fasting (PSMF) is a pattern of eating where you get many of the benefits of fasting (weight loss, improved insulin sensitivity, etc.), without the negatives (loss of lean mass). In a water fast you lose about a third of a pound of lean mass each day of the fast. A 3 day fast during a week results in the loss of a pound of lean mass. Lean mass is not easy to build and we don't want to lose it if we can avoid it.

The idea behind a PSMF is to reduce carbs and fat as much as possible while still hitting your protein goal or even getting a bit more protein than your target. Instead of 0.8 times your lean mass for your protein goal, you want maybe 1.0 times your lean mass when doing a PSMF. The additional protein makes your body use even more stored fat for fuel, helps break stalls or accelerate weight loss and healing, and helps keep you feeling full, while also giving you the added benefit of the high thermic effect of food with protein, which means that you effectively lose 25 percent of the calories you take.

You also want to get some fat during this type of fast to ensure that you keep your hormones happy and that fat-soluble vitamins (A, D, E, and K) get absorbed. 30 to 50 grams of fat will be enough.

THERMIC EFFECT OF FOOD

Thermic effect of food (TEF) is the amount of energy needed to consume and digest different macro nutrients. Some (protein) require much more energy to be consumed than others (carbs and fat). This means that the total calories consumed will result in different amount of effective calories in the body depending on what macro nutrients were consumed.

This chart shows you the thermic effect of different macro nutrients.

Macro Nutrient	Thermic Effect of Food	Calories Consumed	Effective Calories
Fat	3%	100	97
Carbohydrates	8%	100	92
Protein	25%	100	75

Pure Protein Day

In my first book, Secrets to a Healthy Metabolism, I wrote about what I call a "pure protein day." I knew there was a strong thermic effect of food with protein. My guideline for a pure protein day was no carbs (no vegetables, either) and little fat. I was afraid of the backlash from the keto community, so I started calling it a pure protein and fat day. However, now that Craig and I understand the science behind protein-sparing modified fasts, we know that the pure protein day works, and we were right all along!

A pure protein day maintains muscle while you utilize the fat on your body to generate fuel and ketones. The thermic effect of the protein helps burn calories, too!

I often still eat my keto bread (I originally called it "protein bread") with scrambled eggs or a grassfed beef burger.

This chart shows how protein results in more TEF and less effective calories in the body. This is another of the reasons why PSMF are powerful tools for weight loss and forcing the body to consume more bodyfat for fuel which is fat loss.

PSMF EXAMPLE

PSMF is something we treat a bit like water fasting in that we suggest you do it every once in a while—maybe a couple days a week or as needed to break a stall and increase weight loss.

Let's look at an example. A woman that weighs 170 pounds and has 38 percent body fat means she has 105 pounds of lean mass.

$$170 \times 0.38 = 64.6 \text{ pounds of bodyfat}$$

$$170 - 64.6 = 105.4 \text{ pounds of lean mass}$$

$$105 \times 1.0 \text{ is } 105 \text{ grams of protein}$$

Her macros would be little to no carbs, 105 grams of protein, and about 40 grams of fat.

$$40 \text{ grams fat} = 360 \text{ calories (1g fat is 9 calories)}$$

$$360 \text{ minus TEF of } 3\% = 349 \text{ effective calories}$$

$$105 \text{ grams protein} = 420 \text{ calories (1g protein is 4 calories)}$$

$$420 \text{ minus TEF of } 25\% = 315 \text{ effective calories}$$

As you can see, this is like fasting while preserving lean mass because she is only getting about 780 calories, though only about 664 (349+315) of those calories are useful because of the thermic effect of food. She will get enough protein to preserve important lean body mass, but she will have to use a lot of stored fat to fuel her body. This is what makes PSMF such a great tool for accelerating weight loss or breaking a stall.

Being keto adapted before doing PSMF will be very helpful. It is not required but it will make it much easier to do. When you are fully keto adapted (after 4-6 weeks or so) your body will be very efficient at tapping stored bodyfat for fuel. Most of our clients find that PSMF come very easy. The protein is very satiating and they actual stay full throughout the day.

Eight to ten years ago, Maria called this practice a "pure protein day." Back then, we hadn't heard of PSMF. We just knew the properties of the thermic effect of food and how our metabolisms worked, so we knew this could be helpful for people to lose weight faster. PSMF is becoming more popular and well-known and is a great tool for improving results.

So give it a try! You will love the results you see.

> I tried a PSMF ("pure protein day") today... I had to force myself to hit that protein goal, I just wasn't hungry. I used the recommendation from Maria's calculator, and am going to try another one tomorrow... It doesn't feel at all like "fasting"!
>
> —Jillian

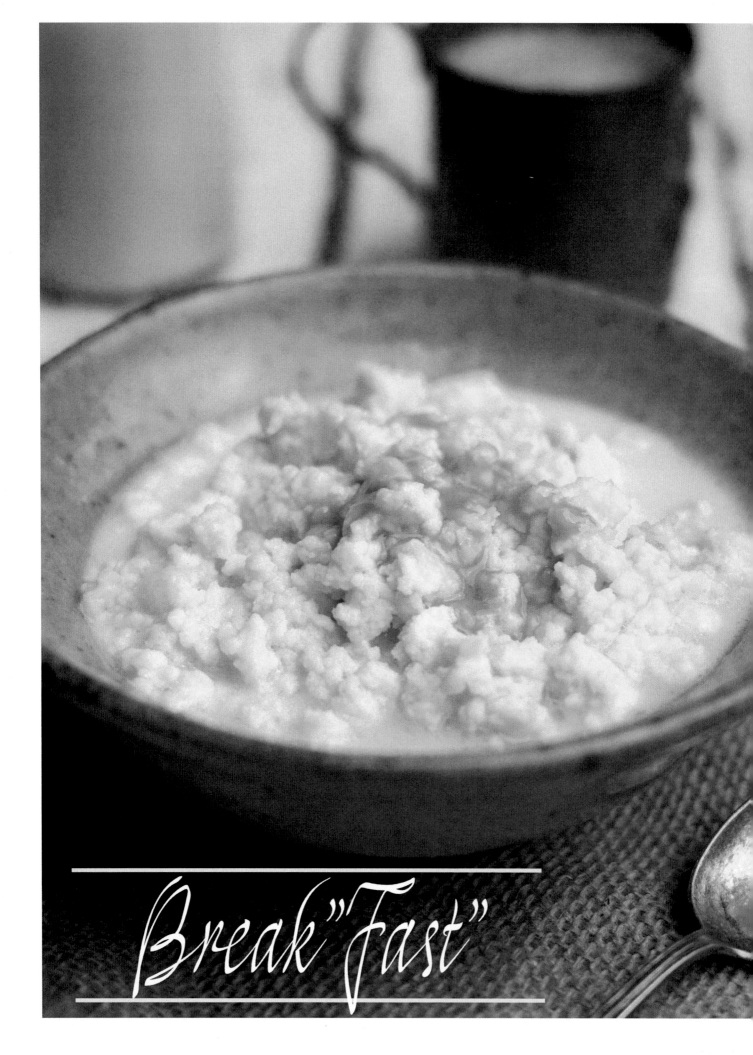

Break"Fast"

French Toast Porridge

Prep Time: 5 minutes
Cook Time: 5 minutes
Servings: 1

8 large egg whites

2/3 cup unsweetened almond milk

a few drops of stevia glycerite to taste

4 teaspoon maple extract

1/2 teaspoon fine sea salt

1 teaspoon butter-flavored coconut oil

Sprinkle of ground cinnamon

1. In a small bowl, whisk together the egg whites, almond milk, sweetener, extract, and salt.

2. In a medium-sized saucepan, melt the oil over medium heat. Add the egg mixture and cook, scraping the bottom with a wooden spoon, until the mixture thickens and starts curdling, about 4 minutes. Use a whisk to help separate the curds.

3. Once the curds form and the mixture has thickened, remove from the heat and transfer to a serving bowl. Sprinkle with cinnamon and serve with ¼ cup unsweetened almond milk if desired.

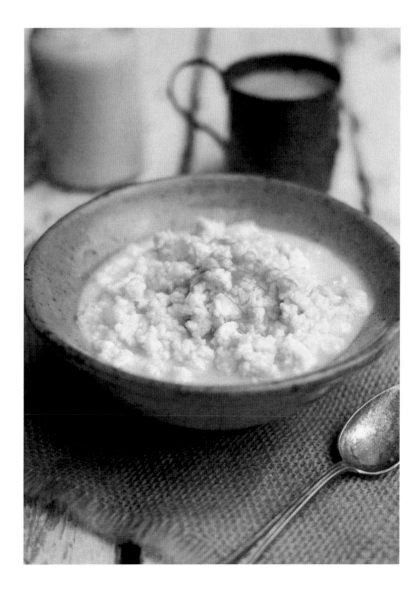

Nutritional Info (per serving)				
Calories	Fat	Protein	Carbs	Fiber
195	7g	29g	2g	0.4g

Chicken Breakfast Patties

Prep Time: 10 minutes
Cook Time: 10 minutes
Servings: 12 (24 total, 2 per)

3 pounds ground chicken or ground turkey

3 teaspoons finely chopped dried sage

2 teaspoons finely chopped dried thyme

1 teaspoon red pepper flakes

½ teaspoon ground nutmeg

1 teaspoon maple extract

¼ teaspoon stevia glycerite

1½ teaspoons fine sea salt

½ teaspoon fresh ground black pepper

1 teaspoon lard or coconut oil, for frying

1. Place all the ingredients and in a large bowl and mix together with your hands until the seasonings are distributed throughout the meat. To check the seasoning, fry up a small dab of the mixture in a skillet over medium heat; taste it and add more seasoning if desired.

2. Form the sausage mixture into twenty-four 2-inch patties.

3. Refrigerate the sausages for a few hours to allow the flavors to meld.

4. Cook within 3 days. Can be frozen for up to a month for easy breakfasts!

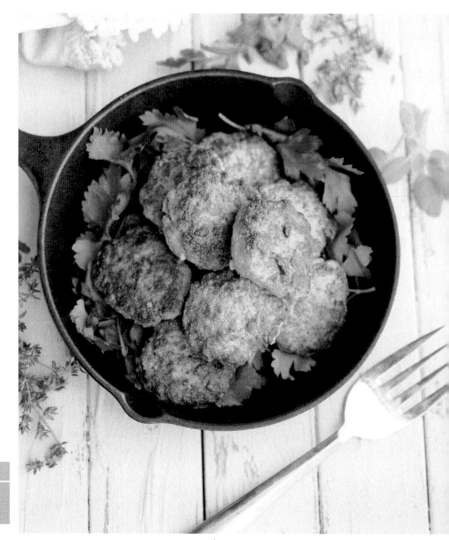

Nutritional Info (per serving)				
Calories	Fat	Protein	Carbs	Fiber
289	16g	31g	3g	1g

Ham Omelet

NUT FREE **DAIRY FREE**

Prep Time: 5 minutes
Cook Time: 10 minutes
Servings: 1

4 large egg whites

1 tablespoon water

⅛ teaspoon fine sea salt

⅛ teaspoon fresh ground black pepper

1 teaspoon butter flavored coconut oil

2 ounce ham, chopped

1. Place the egg whites into a small bowl. Add the water, salt, and pepper and whisk with a fork.

2. Preheat an 8-inch skillet over medium-low heat. Melt the oil in the pan, then pour in the egg mixture and swirl it in the pan. For a few seconds, gently stir the egg mixture with a spatula (as if you were going to make scrambled eggs), then swirl the eggs in the pan to make a nice round shape. Reduce the heat to avoid any color or burning.

3. Continue cooking for about 1 minute. The eggs will be set on the bottom but slightly liquid on top.

4. Remove the pan from the heat. Add the ham to the center of the omelet. Fold the omelet and plate it immediately.

5. Serve with keto bread, if desired.

Nutritional Info (per serving)				
Calories	Fat	Protein	Carbs	Fiber
245	14g	27g	1g	0.1g

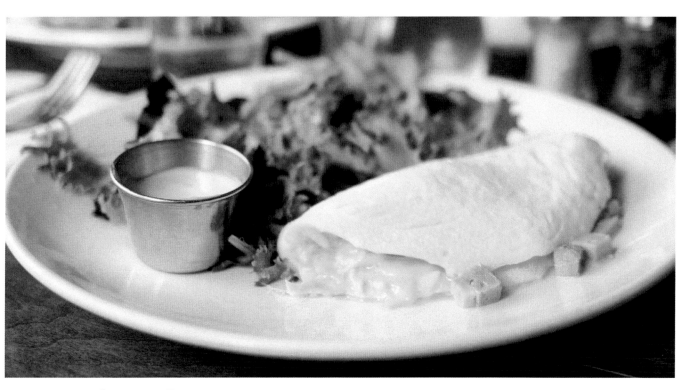

Easy Strawberry Shake

Prep Time: 5 minutes
Cook Time: 0 minutes
Servings: 1

1 cup unsweetened almond milk (or unsweetened Hemp milk if nut free)

1/2 cup beef protein powder or egg white protein powder (check for ZERO carbs)

1 teaspoon Strawberry extract

Few drops strawberry stevia

1   Place everything into a blender and puree until smooth.

Nutritional Info (per serving)				
Calories	Fat	Protein	Carbs	Fiber
203	3g	39g	2g	1g

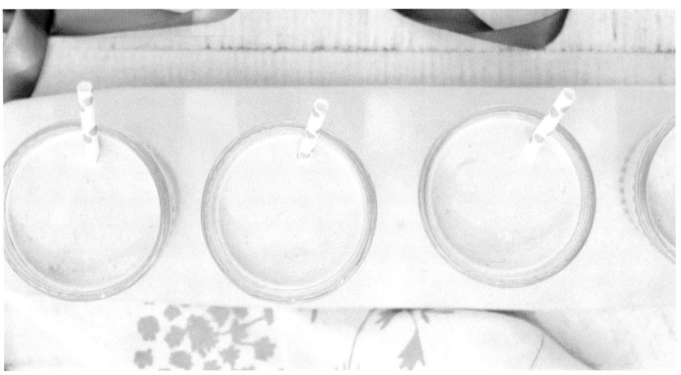

12 - Break"Fast"

Minute Breakfast Muffins

NUT FREE **DAIRY FREE**

Prep Time: 5 minutes
Cook Time: 1-12 minutes
Servings: 2

Coconut oil spray, for the pan

6 slices ham, about 4 inches in diameter

12 egg whites or 6 whole eggs

½ teaspoon fine sea salt

¼ teaspoon fresh ground black pepper

2 tablespoons chopped fresh chives, for garnish

1   Place a slice of ham into a 4 ounce ramekin. Crack 2 egg whites (or 1 whole egg) into the ham in the ramekin. Cover the ramekin with a small plate. Place in microwave for 1 minute or until egg white is cooked through and yolk is a little runny.

2   BAKING OPTION: Preheat the oven to 400°F. Grease a 6-well muffin tin with coconut oil spray. Place 1 slice of ham in each well. Break an egg into each ham cup.

3   Sprinkle the eggs with the salt and pepper. Bake for 12 minutes, or until the egg whites are set but the yolks are still a bit runny.

Nutritional Info (per serving)				
Calories	Fat	Protein	Carbs	Fiber
207	8g	31g	2g	0.2g

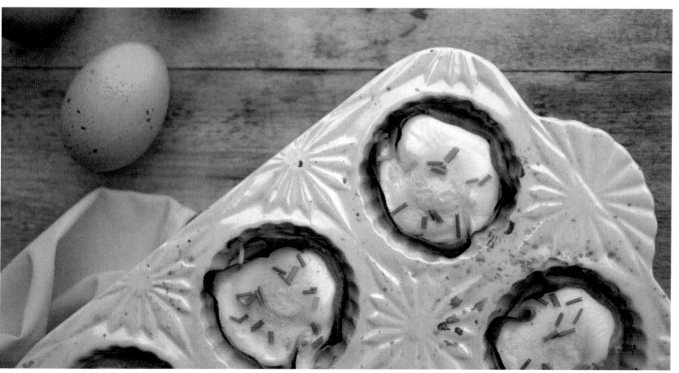

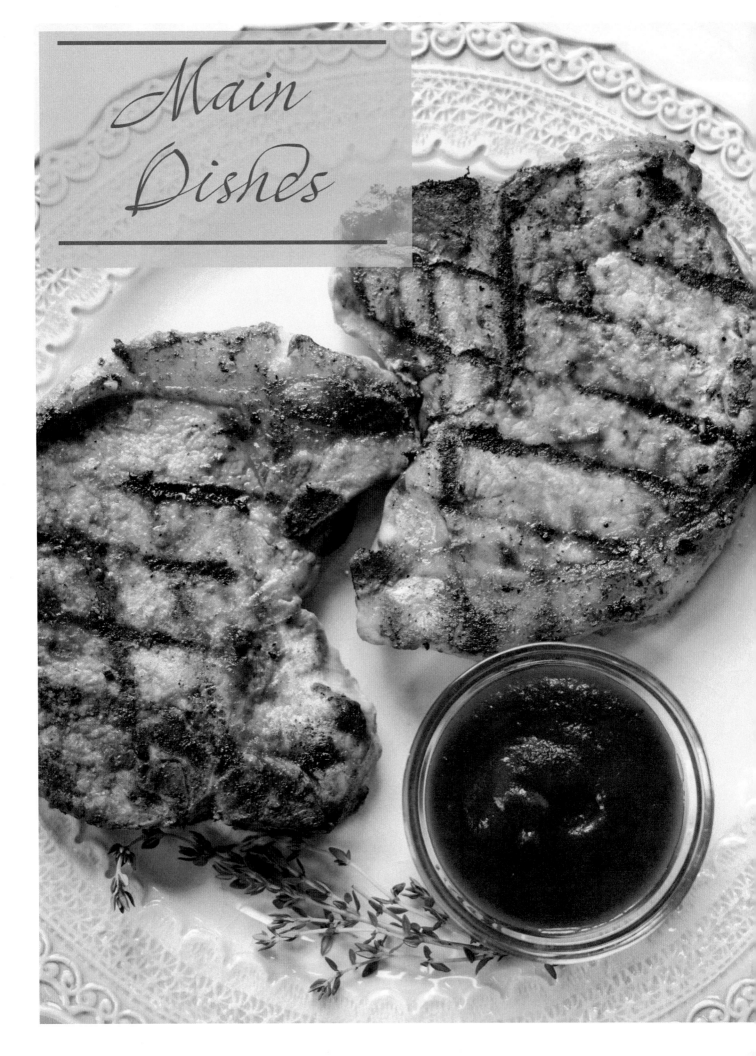

Main
Dishes

Shrimp and Grits

NUT FREE DAIRY FREE

Prep Time: 5 minutes
Cook Time: 12 minutes
Servings: 2

8 large egg whites

1 cup unsweetened almond milk

1 teaspoon fine sea salt

2 teaspoons butter flavored coconut oil, divided

12 precooked large shrimp, cleaned and deveined

1. In a medium-sized bowl, whisk together the eggs, almond milk, and salt.

2. In a large saucepan, melt a teaspoon coconut oil over medium heat. Add the egg mixture to the pan and cook until the mixture thickens and small curds form, all the while scraping the bottom of the pan and stirring to keep large curds from forming. (A whisk works well for this.) This will take about 8 minutes.

3. Meanwhile, heat a large skillet over high heat. Add another teaspoon of oil and, when very hot, season the shrimp with a sprinkle of salt and add them to the pan. Sear for about 20 seconds per side.

4. Place the grits in a serving bowl and top with the seared shrimp. Sprinkle with chopped herbs, if desired, and serve. Best served fresh. Store in an airtight container in the refrigerator for up to 3 days or in the freezer for up to a month. To reheat, place the in a skillet over medium heat for 5 minutes or until warmed through.

Nutritional Info (per serving)				
Calories	Fat	Protein	Carbs	Fiber
191	6g	32g	1g	0.3g

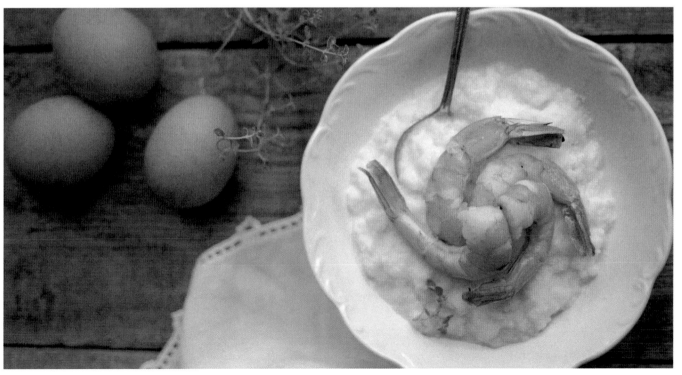

Popovers with Tuna Salad

NUT FREE **DAIRY FREE**

Prep Time: 7 minutes
Cook Time: 25 minutes
Servings: 4

PROTEIN POPOVERS

1/2 cup unflavored EGG WHITE protein powder (do not use whey)

4 TBS coconut oil OR butter, melted (plus extra for greasing)

2 cups unsweetened almond milk

4 eggs

1 teaspoon baking powder

1/2 teaspoon sea salt

TUNA SALAD

2 (5 oz) cans tuna, drained

3 tablespoons mustard

2 tablespoons mayo

¼ teaspoon celery salt (or regular salt)

Fresh ground black pepper

1. Preheat the oven to 425 degree F. Grease popover tins with butter or coconut oil spray. Place the tins in the hot oven for about 8 minutes. Meanwhile, in a medium sized bowl blend together the protein powder, coconut oil, almond milk, eggs, baking powder and salt.

2. Carefully remove hot tin from oven. Dollop 1 tsp of butter or coconut oil into each hot cup and pour the batter in until 2/3 full. Bake for 15 minutes at 425 degree F.

3. POKE HOLES IN THE POPOVERS with a toothpick to release moisture so they don't shrink. Reduce heat to 325 degree F to bake for an additional 10-12 minutes.

4. Meanwhile place the drained tuna, mustard, mayo, celery salt and fresh pepper into a large bowl and combine to coat tuna. Taste and adjust seasoning to your liking.

5. Remove popovers from oven and allow to cool a bit. Serve tuna salad along side the popovers (or slice popovers in ½ and place tuna salad inside each popover). Store in an airtight container in the refrigerator for up to 3 days.

Nutritional Info (per serving)				
Calories	Fat	Protein	Carbs	Fiber
378	26g	34g	1g	0.3g

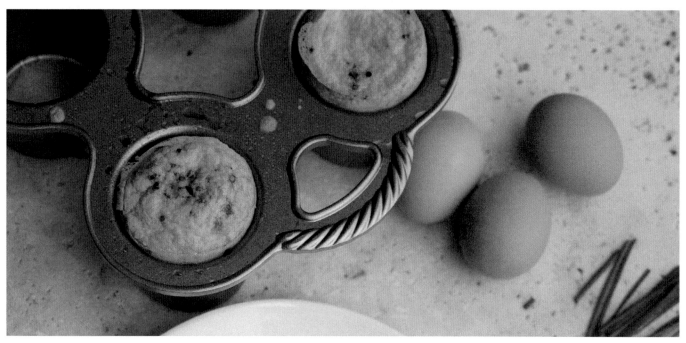

Smoked Chicken Breasts

Prep Time: 10 minutes
Cook Time: 1 1/2 hours
Servings: 8

4 pounds chicken breasts, or drums

1 teaspoon fine sea salt

½ teaspoon ground black pepper

Special equipment:

Smoker

4 cups wood chips of your choice

1   Thirty minutes before you're ready to smoke the chicken, soak the wood chips in water and remove the chicken from the fridge. Season the chicken with the salt and pepper.

2   To smoke the chicken: Read the manufacturer's directions for your smoker before you begin. There are wood, electric, propane, and charcoal smokers, and each type works differently. Start the smoker and if your smoker came with a water bowl, add water to it. When slow cooking meat, it is essential that you have a thermometer to monitor the temperature of the smoker. When the temperature reaches 180°F you can start smoking the chicken.

3   Drain the wood chips and place them into the bottom of the smoker. Place the chicken in the smoker. Secure the lid so it is airtight and no smoke escapes. Smoke the chicken for 30 minutes, and then increase the heat to 230°F. Cook for an additional 45 minutes to 1 hour, or until the internal temperature reaches 165°F. Remove the chicken from the smoker. Cool the chicken and cover it tightly until you're ready to serve it. You can store it in the refrigerator for up to 10 days. If you vacuum-seal it, the smoked chicken will keep for up to 3 weeks.

Nutritional Info (per serving)

Calories	Fat	Protein	Carbs	Fiber
444	17g	67g	0.1g	0g

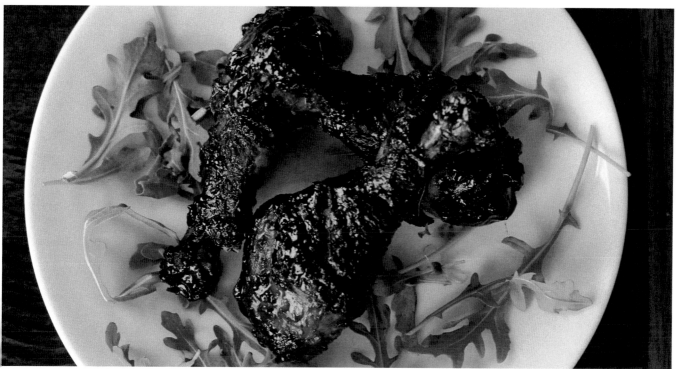

Lean Hamburger Patties
with Mustard

Prep Time: 8 minutes
Cook Time: 6 minutes
Servings: 2

1 pound 95% lean ground beef

2½ teaspoons fine sea salt

1½ teaspoons fresh ground black pepper

1/2 cup Carolina BBQ sauce (or yellow
   mustard) for serving

1 Heat the grill to medium high (or heat 1/2 tablespoon Paleo fat in a cast-iron skillet over medium-high heat).

2 Using your hands, form the meat into 8 patties that are about ½ inch thick. Season the outsides with the salt and pepper. Grill or Fry the burgers in the pan on both sides until they are cooked through, about 3 minutes per side.

3 Remove the burgers from the pan.

4 Serve each burger with Carolina BBQ sauce or mustard. These burgers are best served fresh.

Nutritional Info (per serving)				
Calories	Fat	Protein	Carbs	Fiber
312	11g	49g	1g	0.4g

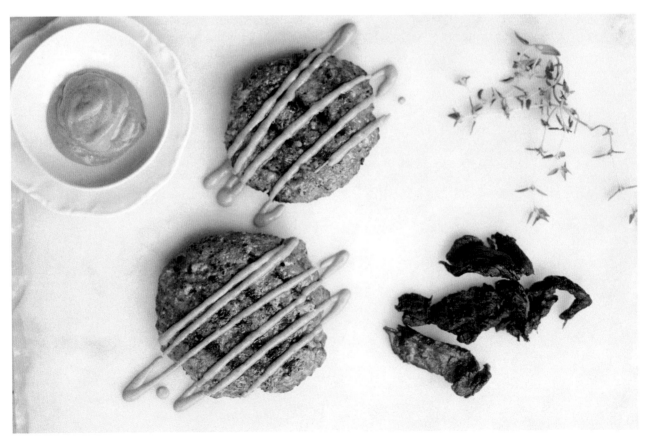

Keto Bread Sandwich

Prep Time: 10 minutes
Cook Time: 40 minutes
Servings: 6

BREAD:

6 large egg whites

¼ cup unflavored egg white protein powder

FILLINGS:

24 slices ham

3 teaspoons Yellow mustard or Carolina BBQ sauce

1   Preheat the oven to 325°F. Grease a 9-by-5-inch loaf pan.

2   Whip the egg whites for a few minutes until very stiff. Slowly fold in the protein powder.

3   Fill the prepared pan with the "dough." Bake for 40 to 45 minutes, until golden brown. Turn oven off and leave in the oven another 10 minutes. Remove from oven and allow to completely cool before cutting or the bread will fall. Cut into 14 slices. Store bread in airtight container in the fridge for up to 6 days. Can be frozen for up to a month.

4   Fill 2 slices with ham and mustard for an easy sandwich.

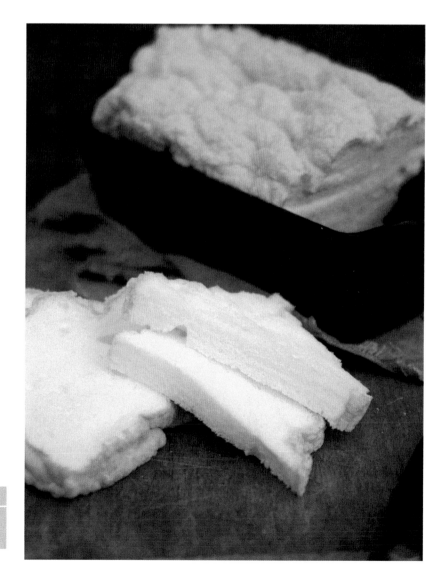

Nutritional Info (per serving)				
Calories	Fat	Protein	Carbs	Fiber
32	0.1g	7g	0.4g	0g

Chicken Fingers
with Carolina BBQ Sauce

Prep Time: 7 minutes
Cook Time: 20 minutes
Servings: 4

1 lemon, sliced thin

4 boneless, skinless chicken breast halves (about 2 pounds), cut into 1-inch-wide strips

2 tablespoons lemon pepper seasoning

2 teaspoons fine sea salt

½ cup Carolina BBQ sauce (page 47)

Chopped fresh parsley and fresh peppercorn (optional), for garnish

1 Preheat the oven to 400°F.

2 Cut lemon into thin slices. Arrange the slices on a rimmed baking sheet or a 13 by 9-inch baking dish.

3 Season all sides of the chicken strips with the lemon pepper seasoning and salt.

4 Bake for 18 to 20 minutes, until the chicken is no longer pink inside. Meanwhile make the Carolina BBQ sauce. Serve with sauce if desired.

5 Store in an airtight container in the refrigerator for up to 3 days or in the freezer for up to a month. To reheat, place the chicken on a rimmed baking sheet in a preheated 375°F oven for 5 minutes or until warmed through.

Nutritional Info (per serving)				
Calories	Fat	Protein	Carbs	Fiber
465	19g	67g	2g	1g

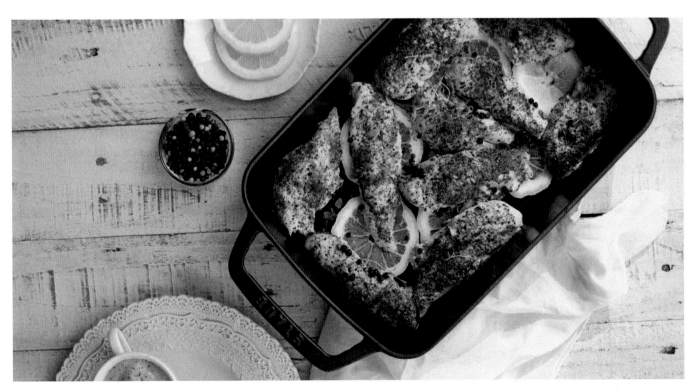

Broiled White Fish with Tartar Sauce

Prep Time: 5 minutes
Cook Time: 10 minutes
Servings: 1

2 (6 ounce) fillets cod (or other white fish)

½ teaspoon fine grain sea salt

½ teaspoon smoked paprika

½ teaspoon garlic powder

½ teaspoon fresh ground pepper

1 ½ tablespoons tartar sauce (page 51)

1   Preheat broiler.

2   Place cod on a cookie sheet with edges. Season fish with salt, paprika, garlic and pepper.

3   Place into oven and broil for 10 minutes or until fish flakes easily with a fork and is cooked through. Serve with a sprinkle of lemon juice if desired.

4   Store in an airtight container in the refrigerator for up to 3 days. To reheat, place on a rimmed baking sheet in a preheated 375°F oven for 5 minutes or until warmed through.

5   Serve with tartar sauce.

Nutritional Info (per serving)				
Calories	Fat	Protein	Carbs	Fiber
285	10g	43g	3g	1g

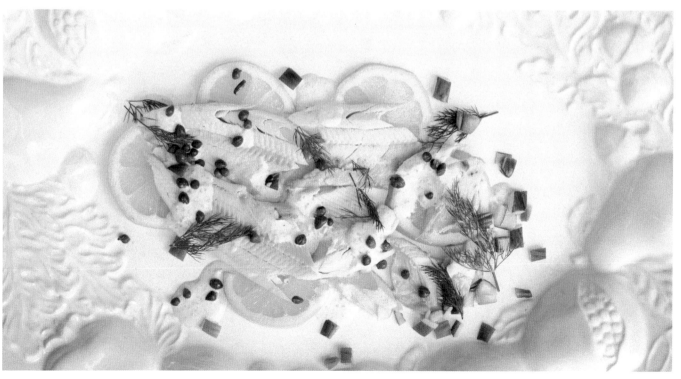

Instant Pot or Slow Cooker Shredded Pork Loin

NUT FREE   DAIRY FREE

Prep Time: 5 minutes
Cook Time: 60 min IP, 8 hours SC
Servings: 8

4 lbs boneless pork loin

5 cloves fresh garlic, sliced

¼ cup diced onion

2 c. chicken broth or store bought

1/2 cup tomato sauce

2 tsp liquid smoke

2 TBS smoky paprika

1 1/2 tsp chili powder

1 tsp Celtic sea salt

1 tsp freshly ground pepper

1   Using a sharp paring knife, cut deep slits in the meat and push slices of garlic inside the slits.

2   INSTANT POT: Place the roast in a 6 quart Instant Pot. Add the onions, broth, liquid smoke, paprika, chili powder, salt and fresh black pepper into the pot. Seal and press Manual to bake for 60 minutes. Once finished, press Natural Release.

3   NOTE: If your pork shoulder roast is only 4 pounds cook on Manual for 45 minutes.

4   SLOW COOKER: Place roast in a 4-quart slow cooker. Add the rest of the ingredients. Cover and cook on low for 8 hours (test with a meat thermometer to make sure it reads 160 degrees F).

5   SERVE: Shred with 2 forks and serve.

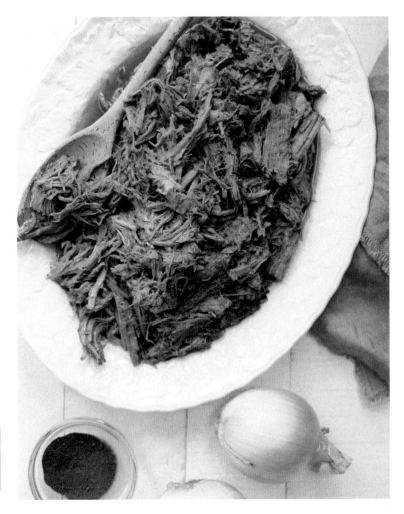

Nutritional Info (per serving)				
Calories	Fat	Protein	Carbs	Fiber
313	10g	49g	5g	2g

Slow Cooker Shredded Ranch Chicken

Prep Time: 5 minutes
Cook Time: 6-8 hours
Servings: 8

4 6-ounce boneless skinless chicken breasts

1 cup chicken broth (preferably kettle and fire organic fat free)

2 tablespoons dried parsley

1 tablespoon onion powder

2 teaspoons garlic powder

1½ teaspoons dried dill weed

1 teaspoon dried chives

1 teaspoon fine sea salt

1 teaspoon fresh ground black pepper

1   Place all the ingredients in a 4 quart slow cooker. Turn on low for 6-8 hours (or on high for 4 hours). Shred with a fork. Serve with leftover sauce in the slow cooker.

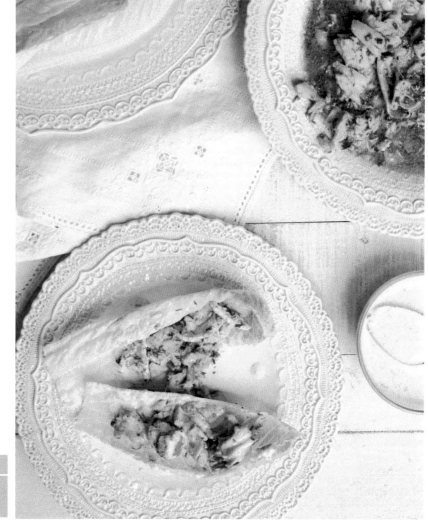

Nutritional Info (per serving)				
Calories	Fat	Protein	Carbs	Fiber
361	15g	52g	2g	1g

Chicken Soup

Prep Time: 8 minutes
Cook Time: 13 minutes
Servings: 4

1 tablespoon butter-flavored coconut oil (or lard)

¼ cup diced onions

2 cloves garlic, crushed to a paste

3 boneless, skinless chicken breasts, 18 ounces cubed into 1 inch pieces

8 cups chicken broth

Fine sea salt and fresh ground black pepper

Fresh thyme leaves or other herb such as parsley or cilantro, for garnish

1   Heat the coconut oil or lard in a large pot over medium heat. Add the onions and garlic and sauté for 5 minutes, or until the onion is translucent. Add the diced chicken to the pot and saute for 5 minutes, or until the chicken is cooked through and no longer pink inside. Add the broth and the herbs and bring to a simmer for 3 minutes.

2   Divide the soup among four bowls and garnish with fresh herbs.

3   Store extras in airtight containers in the fridge for up to 4 days or in the freezer for up to a month. To reheat, place in a saucepot over medium heat for 5 minutes or until heated through.

Nutritional Info (per serving)				
Calories	Fat	Protein	Carbs	Fiber
386	15g	58g	2g	0.3g

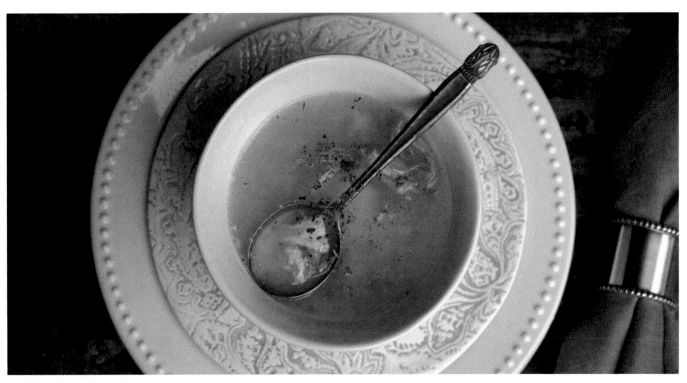

PerfectTenderloin

Prep Time: 5 minutes
Cook Time: 40 minutes
Servings: 8

2 (2-pound) pork tenderloins

8 cloves garlic, sliced in half lengthwise

2 tablespoons wheat-free tamari

2 tablespoons lime juice

1 tablespoon peeled and grated fresh ginger

1 teaspoon stevia glycerite (or a few drops liquid stevia)

4 drops orange oil (optional)

For Garnish (optional):

Chopped fresh cilantro

Lime slices

1   Preheat the oven to 350°F.

2   Place the tenderloins in the baking dish, then cut 16 small slits into the top of each loin, just deep enough to fit half a clove of garlic. Push the garlic into the slits.

3   Place the tamari, lime juice, ginger, stevia and orange oil, if using, in a small bowl and stir well to combine. Pour over the pork in the baking dish.

4   Bake for 40 minutes or until the pork is cooked through and no longer pink inside. (A meat thermometer should read 140°F when inserted into the middle of one of the tenderloins.)

5   Place the pork on a cutting board to rest for 10 minutes before slicing. Cut into ½-inch slices and pour the sauce from the pan over the pork. Garnish with cilantro and lime slices, if desired.

6   Store in an airtight container in the refrigerator for up to 4 days. To reheat, place the pork in a baking dish in a preheated 350°F oven for 4 minutes or until warmed through.

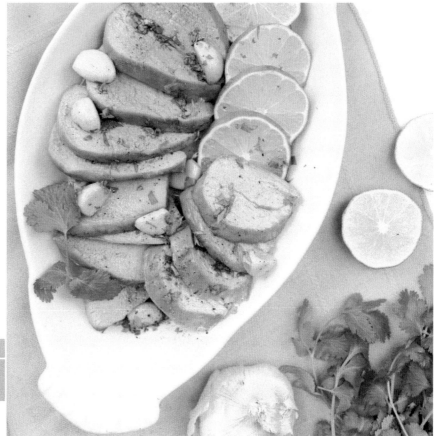

Nutritional Info (per serving)				
Calories	Fat	Protein	Carbs	Fiber
324	13g	47g	2g	0.1g

Perfect Pork Chop with Dijon vinegar

Prep Time: 10 minutes
Cook Time: 15 minutes
Servings: 4

1 tablespoon lard

4 (5-ounce) bone-in pork chops, about ¾ inch thick with visible fat removed

Fine sea salt and fresh ground black pepper

8 tablespoons Dijon Vinaigrette (page 48)

1 Preheat a large cast-iron skillet over medium-high heat; once hot, place the lard in the pan. While the pan is heating, prepare the chops: pat the pork chops dry and season both sides liberally with salt and pepper.

2 When the fat is hot, place the chops in the skillet and sear for about 3½ minutes, then flip them over and sear the other side until the chops are cooked through, about 3½ more minutes (the cooking time will depend on the thickness of the chops). Do not overcrowd the pan; if necessary, cook the chops in batches

3 Remove chops from the pan and set aside to rest. Place the Dijon in the skillet with the drippings. Slowly whisk the vinegar and broth and whisk to combine. Bring to a simmer and boil to reduce a little and remove from heat. Add thyme, salt and pepper to taste. Serve chops with the sauce. Garnish with fresh thyme leaves if desired.

4 Store extras in an airtight container in the fridge for up to 3 days. To reheat, place the chops in a skillet over medium heat and sauté for 3 minutes per side, or until warmed.

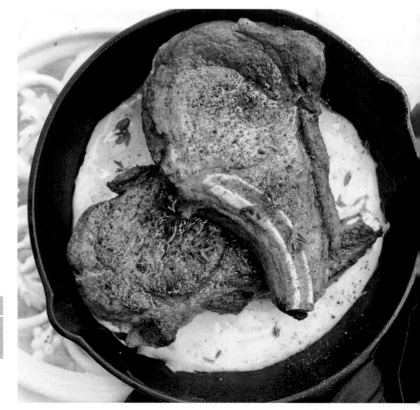

Nutritional Info (per serving)				
Calories	Fat	Protein	Carbs	Fiber
381	23g	36g	2g	0.2g

Lobster Tails

NUT FREE DAIRY FREE

Prep Time: 5 minutes
Cook Time: 10 minutes
Servings: 1

2 4-ounce lobster tails, thawed

Salt for poaching water

Optional Sauce for serving: Carolina BBQ
    sauce (page 47), or Dijon Vinaigrette
    (page 48)

1   Fill a pot with enough water to cover up to 2 tails. Add 2 tablespoons salt to the water. Bring the water to a boil and gently drop tails into the pot. Once the tails have been placed in the pot, wait for the water to reach a slow boil, then reduce the heat and simmer uncovered for 3-½ minutes.

2   Remove all tails from the pot, but keep the water on the stove at a slow boil in case you need to boil it longer. After removing the tails from the pot, allow to cool down a little, and then test just one tail for doneness.

3   Use a knife to cut through the soft underside of the shell and into the thickest part of the tail meat. If it appears completely white with no signs of translucent, grayish coloring, then your boiled lobster tails are ready to serve.

4   Serve with optional sauce if desired. Best served fresh.

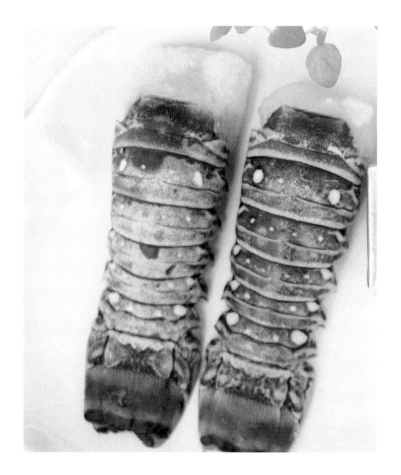

Nutritional Info (per serving)

Calories	Fat	Protein	Carbs	Fiber
225	3g	48g	0g	0g

Grilled Fillet Mignon

Prep Time: 5 minutes
Cook Time: 15 minutes
Servings: 1

2 (3-ounce) filet mignons

Fine sea salt and ground black pepper

1 Season the filets well on all sides with salt and pepper. Let sit at room temperature for 15 minutes.

2 Heat a grill to medium-high heat.

3 Once hot, add the filets and sear on both sides until cooked to your desired doneness (see chart below).

4 Remove the filets from the skillet and allow them to rest for 10 minutes. This dish is best served fresh.

Doneness Chart:

Rare: 120°F to 125°F

Medium-rare: 130°F to 135°F

Medium: 140°F to 145°F

Medium-well: 150°F to 155°F

Nutritional Info (per serving)				
Calories	Fat	Protein	Carbs	Fiber
250	11g	35g	0g	0g

Canned Tuna with Dijon Mustard

Prep Time: 7 minutes
Cook Time: 0 minutes
Servings: 2

2 (5 oz) cans tuna, drained

4 tablespoons Dijon mustard

¼ teaspoon celery salt (or regular salt)

Fresh ground black pepper

1 Place the drained tuna, mustard, celery salt and fresh pepper into a large bowl and combine to coat tuna. Taste and adjust seasoning to your liking.

2 Store in an airtight container in the refrigerator for up to 4 days.

Nutritional Info (per serving)				
Calories	Fat	Protein	Carbs	Fiber
196	1g	36g	0.3g	0.1g

Crab Legs with Spicy Mustard

NUT FREE   DAIRY FREE

Prep Time: 5 minutes
Cook Time: 3 minutes
Servings: 4

Fine sea salt

12 medium Alaskan king crab legs, thawed

Spicy Mustard Sauce:

1/2 cup Dijon mustard

2 tablespoons mayo

1 tablespoon prepared horseradish

2 teaspoons lime or lemon juice

2 or 3 drops hot sauce

Fine sea salt (optional)

For Garnish (optional):

Lime wedges

Fresh parsley

1 Fill a large stockpot about two-thirds full with water. Add about 2 tablespoons of salt to the water and bring to a boil. Add the crab claws and boil for 3 minutes or until warmed through.

2 Meanwhile, make the sauce: Place the mayo, mustard, horseradish, lime juice, and hot sauce in a small bowl. Stir well to combine. Taste and add salt, if needed.

3 Place the crab claws on a platter and serve with a bowl of the spicy mustard sauce. Garnish the platter with lime wedges and parsley, if desired.

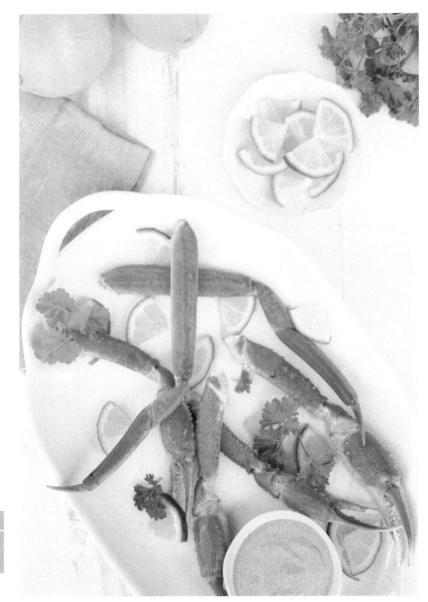

Nutritional Info (per serving)				
Calories	Fat	Protein	Carbs	Fiber
374	8g	71g	1g	0.2g

29 - Main

Simple Poached Turkey Breast

Prep Time: 7 minutes
Cook Time: 90 minutes
Servings: 8

1/4 cup Dijon mustard

1 clove garlic, minced

1 teaspoon paprika

1 teaspoon Italian seasoning

1/2 teaspoon fine grain sea salt

1 (3 pound) skinless turkey breast

1 Preheat oven to 350 degrees F (175 degrees C).

2 Mix 1/4 cup Dijon, garlic, paprika, Italian seasoning, salt, and black pepper in a bowl. Place turkey breast into a roasting pan. Brush half the Dijon mixture over the turkey breast. Reserve remaining Dijon mixture. Tent turkey breast loosely with aluminum foil.

3 Roast in the preheated oven for 1 hour; baste turkey breast with more Dijon mixture. Return to oven and roast until the juices run clear and an instant-read meat thermometer inserted into the thickest part of the breast, not touching bone, reads 165 degrees F (65 degrees C), about 15-25 more minutes. Let turkey breast rest 10 to 15 minutes before serving. Serve with extra sauce if desired.

Nutritional Info (per serving)				
Calories	Fat	Protein	Carbs	Fiber
257	4g	52g	0.1g	0g

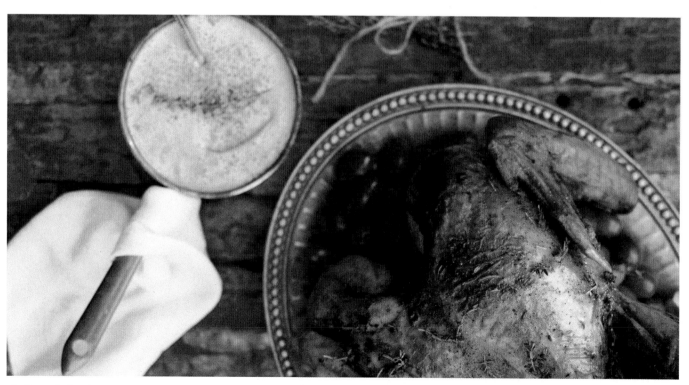

Grilled Chicken Breasts with Carolina BBQ Sauce

NUT FREE DAIRY FREE

Prep Time: 7 minutes
Cook Time: 10 minutes
Servings: 4

4 boneless skinless chicken breasts

2 teaspoons Fine grain sea salt

2 teaspoons Freshly ground black pepper

½ teaspoon garlic powder

½ cup Carolina BBQ sauce (page 47)

1 Preheat grill on high, 5 minutes. Season chicken generously with salt and pepper. Using long tongs, place chicken breasts on grill and cook, covered on high, 3 minutes. Flip breasts and continue cooking on high, 3 more minutes.

2 Reduce grill heat to low and flip chicken again. Flip chicken again and cook 3 more minutes on low, or until a meat thermometer reads 160° when inserted into the thickest part of the meat. Meanwhile make the Carolina BBQ sauce (page 47).

3 To serve, remove chicken and drizzle with Carolina BBQ sauce.

4 Store extras in airtight container in the fridge for up to 5 days. Can be served warm or cold.

Nutritional Info (per serving)				
Calories	Fat	Protein	Carbs	Fiber
304	13g	43g	2g	1g

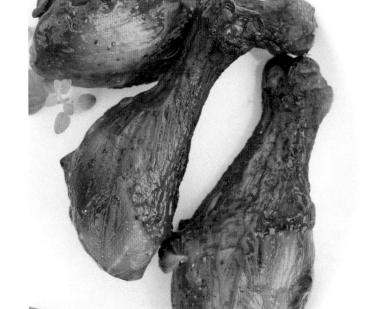

Keto Fried Rice with Ground Chicken

NUT FREE **DAIRY FREE**

Prep Time: 5 minutes
Cook Time: 15 minutes
Servings: 4

12 large egg whites

½ cup beef bone broth, homemade or store-bought

2 teaspoons wheat-free tamari, or 3 teaspoons coconut aminos

1 teaspoon fine sea salt

½ teaspoon ground black pepper

1 teaspoon lard or coconut oil

¼ cup diced onions

1 clove garlic, minced

1 pound lean ground turkey or ground chicken

For Garnish (optional):

1 teaspoon crushed red pepper

Thinly sliced scallions

1. Place egg whites medium-sized bowl. Add the broth, tamari, salt, and pepper and whisk until well combined.

2. In a large skillet over medium heat, place a teaspoon of lard or coconut oil. Add the onions and garlic to the skillet and sauté until the onions are translucent, about 2 minutes. Place the ground turkey to the skillet. Cook for 2 minutes and season well with salt and pepper.

3. Pour the egg mixture into the skillet and cook until the mixture thickens and small curds form, while scraping the bottom of the pan and whisking to keep large curds from forming. (A whisk works well for this task.) This will take about 7 minutes.

4. Place the "fried rice" on a platter. Garnish with crushed red pepper and scallions, if desired, and serve.

5. Store in an airtight container in the refrigerator for up to 3 days. To reheat, place the shrimp fried "rice" in a lightly greased sauté pan over medium heat, stirring often, for 2 minutes or until warmed through.

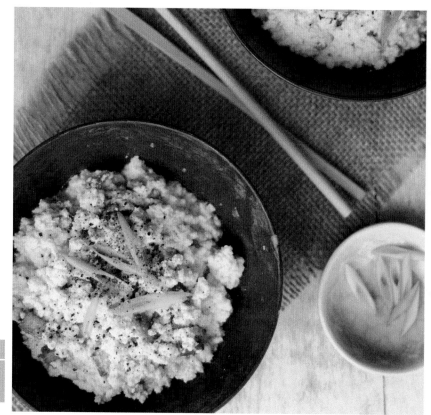

Nutritional Info (per serving)				
Calories	Fat	Protein	Carbs	Fiber
341	17g	42g	2g	0.2g

Surf and Turf with Carolina BBQ Sauce

NUT FREE **DAIRY FREE**

Prep Time: 5 minutes
Cook Time: 15 minutes
Servings: 2

2 (3-ounce) filet mignons

Fine sea salt and ground black pepper

4 jumbo prawns or jumbo shrimp, shell-on, butterflied and deveined

2 tablespoons keto fat of choice, for frying

¼ cup Carolina BBQ sauce (page 47)

Steak Doneness Chart:

Rare: 120°F to 125°F

Medium-rare: 130°F to 135°F

Medium: 140°F to 145°F

Medium-well: 150°F to 155°F

1. Season the filets well on all sides with salt and pepper. Let sit at room temperature for 15 minutes.

2. Heat a cast-iron skillet over medium-high heat. Season the prawns well with salt and pepper.

3. Melt the fat in the hot pan, then add the filets and sear on both sides until cooked to your desired doneness (see chart below).

4. Remove the filets from the skillet and allow them to rest for 10 minutes. While the filets are resting, fry the prawns in the same skillet until the shells have turned pink and the meat is cooked through and no longer translucent, about 3 minutes per side.

5. Place each steak on a plate. Top with a prawn and drizzle each plate with 2 tablespoons of the sauce. This dish is best served fresh.

Nutritional Info (per serving)				
Calories	Fat	Protein	Carbs	Fiber
316	22g	29g	2g	1g

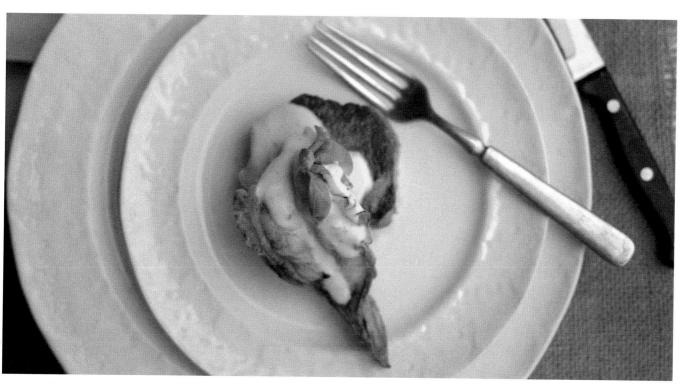

Broiled Shrimp with Cilantro Lime Sauce

Prep Time: 8 minutes
Cook Time: 5 minutes
Servings: 1

2 tablespoons avocado oil or melted coconut oil

1 tablespoon lime or lemon juice

1 teaspoon fine grain sea salt

1 teaspoon paprika

1 clove garlic, smashed

½ pound peeled and cleaned shrimp

¼ cup Cilantro Sauce: (see page 49)

1 Preheat broiler. Place oil, lime juice, salt, paprika, and smashed garlic in a large bowl. Stir well to combine. Add peeled shrimp and stir well to combine all over shrimp. Place on baking sheet with edges and broil for 5 minutes or until shrimp is cooked through.

2 Meanwhile make the sauce. Serve along side shrimp for dipping.

Nutritional Info (per serving)				
Calories	Fat	Protein	Carbs	Fiber
274	14g	35g	4g	0.4g

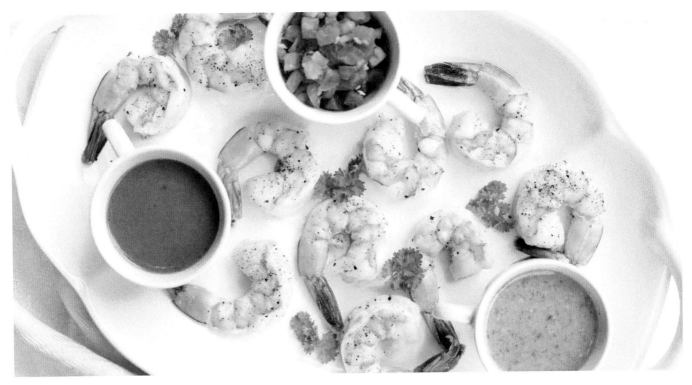

Fried Soft Shell Crab

NUT FREE DAIRY FREE

Prep Time: 8 minutes
Cook Time: 8 minutes
Servings: 2

8 soft shell crabs (2 Sizzlefish packages)

1/2 cup powdered Parmesan (I put shredded Parmesan in a food processor and pureed until smooth) or powdered pork rinds for dairy free

2 eggs, beaten

4 tablespoons Carolina BBQ sauce (page 47)

1 Heat a cast iron skillet with 1/2 cup lard or tallow to medium high heat. Pat the crab dry with paper towel. Place the powdered parmesan into a large shallow dish. Place the beaten eggs into another large shallow dish.

2 Dip the crab into the eggs and tap, just so the crab has a light coating. Dip into the parmesan and use your hands to coat the crab well.

3 Drop 3-4 crabs into the hot oil and cook for 2 minutes, flip and cook another 2 minutes or until crab is cooked through.

4 Repeat with remaining crabs.

5 While the crab cooks, prepare my Carolina BBQ sauce and serve with delicious crispy crab! Best served fresh.

Nutritional Info (per serving)				
Calories	Fat	Protein	Carbs	Fiber
388	14g	60g	2g	1g

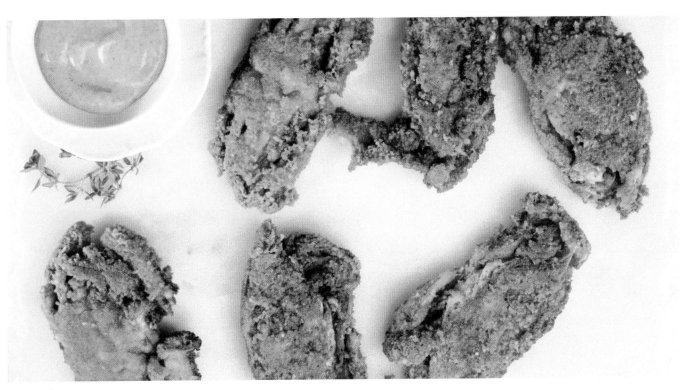

BBQ Pork Chops

Prep Time: 5 minutes
Cook Time: 7 minutes
Servings: 4

4 (5-ounce) bone-in pork chops, about ¾ inch thick

Fine sea salt and fresh ground black pepper

1/2 cup Keto BBQ Sauce (page 50), or AlternaSweets BBQ Sauce

1   Preheat grill to medium-high heat. While the grill is heating, prepare the chops: pat the pork chops dry and season both sides liberally with salt and pepper.

2   When the grill is hot, place the chops on the grill and cook for about 3½ minutes, then flip them over and sear the other side until the chops are cooked through, about 3½ more minutes (the cooking time will depend on the thickness of the chops). Meanwhile make the BBQ sauce or get out the AlternaSweets sugar free BBQ sauce.

3   Brush chops with BBQ sauce and cook a few more seconds. Brush the other side and grill a few more seconds. Remove from grill and serve with extra BBQ Sauce.

4   Store extras in an airtight container in the fridge for up to 3 days. To reheat, place the chops and kraut in a skillet over medium heat and sauté for 3 minutes per side, or until warmed.

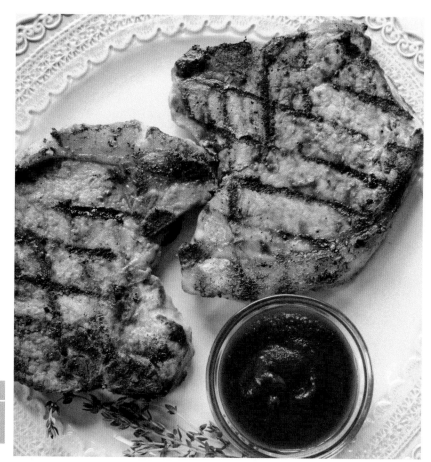

Nutritional Info (per serving)				
Calories	Fat	Protein	Carbs	Fiber
301	19g	28g	2g	1g

Mojito Chicken

NUT FREE   DAIRY FREE

Prep Time: 7 minutes
Cook Time: 30 minutes
Servings: 6

Marinade:

3/4 cup fresh lime juice

1/2 cup MCT oil or avocado oil

1/2 cup finely chopped fresh mint

2 teaspoons smashed garlic

1 tablespoon fine grain sea salt

6 chicken legs or thighs

Garnish:

2 small limes, sliced thin or quartered

Fresh mint leaves

1   Place lime juice, oil, mint, garlic and salt in a large shallow baking dish. Add chicken and roll around to coat well. Cover and chill for 3 hours or overnight.

2   Heat grill to medium heat. Place chicken onto the grill. Discard extra marinade. Cook chicken for 15 minutes per side or until cooked through and no longer pink inside. Place onto a serving platter. Garnish chicken with slices of lime and fresh mint. Squeeze limes over chicken and serve.

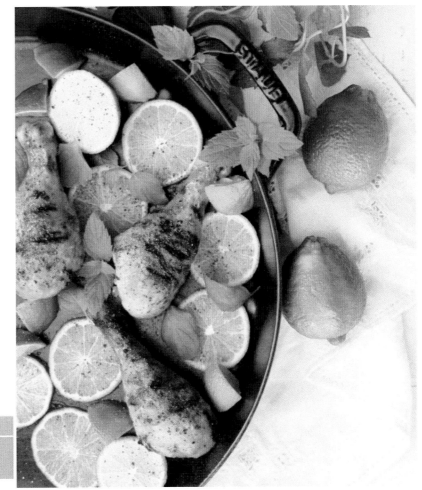

Nutritional Info (per serving)				
Calories	Fat	Protein	Carbs	Fiber
282	17g	29g	1g	0.1g

Simple Shrimp Adobo

Prep Time: 5 minutes
Cook Time: 4 minutes
Servings: 2

1 pound medium shrimp, peeled and cleaned

1/4 cup Coconut Vinegar

1/4 cup organic tamari sauce

2 tablespoons lime juice

2 tablespoons Peppercorns

1 teaspoon fine grain sea Salt

1 teaspoon fish sauce (or more salt)

2 cloves Garlic, minced

2 tablespoons coconut Oil or ghee

1   Place shrimp into a large bowl. Add vinegar, coconut aminos, lime juice, peppercorns, salt, fish sauce and garlic.

2   Place oil in a large wok or cast iron skillet. Heat to medium high. One the oil is hot, add the shrimp along with the marinade. Stir-fry and cook for 5 minutes, or until shrimp are cooked through and no longer opaque.

Nutritional Info (per serving)				
Calories	Fat	Protein	Carbs	Fiber
287	14g	39g	4g	0.2g

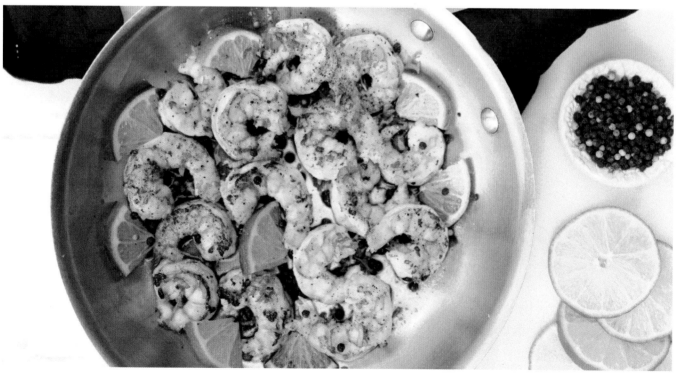

Indian Shrimp over Keto Rice

NUT FREE **DAIRY FREE**

Prep Time: 8 minutes
Cook Time: 10 minutes
Servings: 8

¼ cup coconut oil

1/2 cup diced onions

6 cloves garlic, minced

2 tablespoons fresh grated ginger

2 pounds shrimp, peeled and deveined

4 tablespoons chicken bone broth
   (homemade or boxed)

3 tablespoons garam masala

2 tablespoons yellow curry paste

1 tablespoon ground turmeric

2 teaspoons fine grain sea salt

1 tablespoon lime juice

Garnish with fresh cilantro and green
   onion sliced on the diagonal

1 batch Keto Fried Rice for serving

1 Place the coconut oil in a large cast iron skillet to medium high. Add onions and sauté for 3 minutes or until onions are soft. Add garlic and ginger and sauté another 2 minutes. Season shrimp on all sides with salt and cook in the skillet on each side for 2 minutes or until cooked through and no longer translucent. Add broth, garam masala, curry paste and ground turmeric. Stir until well mixed.

2 Simmer over medium for 2 minutes. Add lime juice and stir garnish with sliced limes, cilantro and green onion. Serve over keto fried rice. Store extras in an airtight container in the refrigerator for up to 3 days. To reheat, place in a lightly greased sauté pan

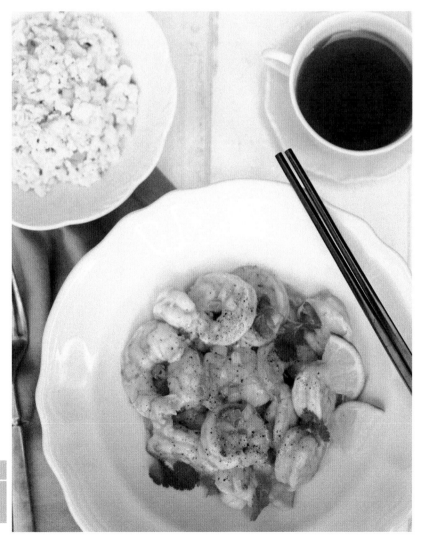

Nutritional Info (per serving)				
Calories	Fat	Protein	Carbs	Fiber
252	15g	24g	6g	1g

Shrimp Fried Rice

Prep Time: 5 minutes
Cook Time: 15 minutes
Servings: 4

12 egg whites

½ cup beef bone broth, homemade or storebought

2 teaspoons wheat-free tamari, or 3 teaspoons coconut aminos

1 teaspoon fine sea salt

½ teaspoon ground black pepper

3 strips bacon, diced

¼ cup diced onions

1 clove garlic, minced

1 pound large shrimp, peeled and deveined

For Garnish (optional):

1 teaspoon crushed red pepper

Thinly sliced scallions

1 Place egg whites into a medium-sized bowl. Add the broth, tamari, salt, and pepper and whisk until well combined.

2 In a large skillet over medium heat, cook the bacon until crisp, about 4 minutes. Using a slotted spoon, remove the bacon; leave the drippings in the pan. Add the onions and garlic to the skillet and sauté until the onions are translucent, about 2 minutes. Season the shrimp on all sides with salt and pepper and add to the skillet. Cook for 2 minutes on each side.

3 Make the "rice": Pour the egg mixture into the skillet and cook until the mixture thickens and small curds form, while scraping the bottom of the pan and whisking to keep large curds from forming. (A whisk works well for this task.) This will take about 7 minutes. Stir in the reserved bacon.

4 Place the "rice" on a platter. Garnish with crushed red pepper and scallions, if desired, and serve.

5 Store in an airtight container in the refrigerator for up to 3 days. To reheat, place the shrimp fried "rice" in a lightly greased sauté pan over medium heat, stirring often, for 2 minutes or until warmed through.

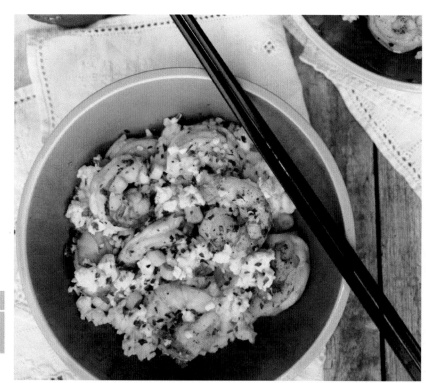

Nutritional Info (per serving)				
Calories	Fat	Protein	Carbs	Fiber
183	5g	32g	2g	0.2g

BBQ Grilled Chicken

Prep Time: 7 minutes
Cook Time: 30 minutes
Servings: 3

6 chicken legs or thighs

1/2 tablespoon fine grain sea salt

1 teaspoon smoked paprika

1/2 cup AlternaSweets BBQ Sauce

1   Heat grill to medium heat. Pat the chicken legs dry. Season chicken on all sides with salt and paprika. Place chicken onto the grill and cook for 15 minutes per side or until cooked through and no longer pink inside. Internal temperature should be 185 degrees F. Brush chicken with BBQ sauce and grill another 30 seconds. Place onto a serving platter. Garnish chicken with additional BBQ sauce.

I highly suggest that you do not skip the step of patting the chicken dry or you will not have crispy skin.

Nutritional Info (per serving)				
Calories	Fat	Protein	Carbs	Fiber
534	30g	59g	3g	1g

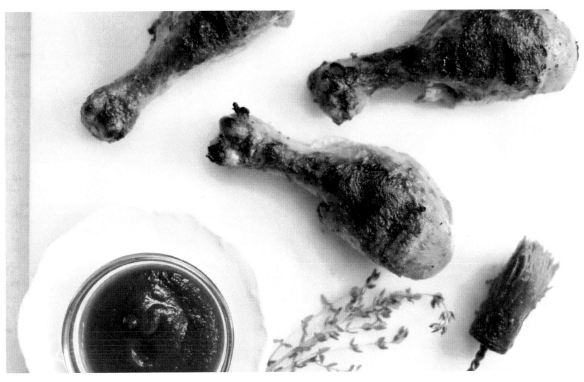

Salt-Crusted Fish

Prep Time: 7 minutes
Cook Time: 25 minutes
Servings: 4

2 tablespoons fresh herbs, such as parsley
    or thyme

1 lemon, thinly sliced

1 (3-pound) whole trout, gutted, gills and
    fins removed

4 large egg whites

2 cups coarse sea salt

For Garnish:

2 tablespoons fresh dill

2 tablespoons capers

1 Preheat the oven to 450°F.

2 Place the herbs and lemon slices inside the body of the fish. Set aside.

3 Place the egg whites in a mixing bowl or the bowl of a stand mixer. Whisk until soft peaks form. Gently fold the salt into the whites with a spatula.

4 Place about ¼ cup of the egg white mixture on an ovenproof platter. Spread the mixture into the size and shape of the trout. Place the trout on top of the mixture, then top the trout with the rest of the egg white mixture, covering it completely. Place the platter on a rimmed baking sheet and bake for 25 minutes or until the fish is no longer opaque and flakes easily with a fork.

5 Let the fish rest for 10 minutes. For a dramatic presentation, move the platter to the dinner table and crack the salt crust open in front of your guests. Then place pieces of fish on serving plates and garnish with diced red onions, fresh dill, capers, and lemon slices.

6 Store in an airtight container in the refrigerator for up to 3 days. To reheat, place the fish in a baking dish in a preheated 350°F oven for 5 minutes or until warmed through.

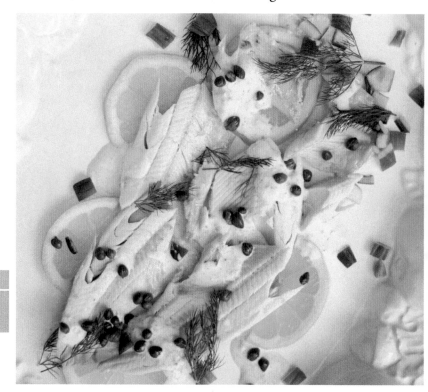

Nutritional Info (per serving)				
Calories	Fat	Protein	Carbs	Fiber
494	19g	75g	2g	1g

Asian Ground Turkey

Prep Time: 5 minutes
Cook Time: 5 minutes
Servings: 3

1/2 tablespoon toasted sesame oil

3 garlic cloves, minced

1 green onion, sliced

1 lb ground turkey or chicken

1/2 teaspoon fine grain sea salt

1/2 teaspoon fresh ground pepper

2 tablespoons tamari sauce

1 teaspoon stevia glycerite or ha1/4
   teaspoon liquid stevia

1 teaspoon minced ginger

1 teaspoon white vinegar

Red pepper flakes, to desired heat

1 Place oil in a large skillet and heat to medium heat. Add garlic and onions and sauté for 1 minute. Add the ground turkey, salt, pepper, tamari, stevia, ginger, vinegar and red pepper flakes if desired. Cook while crumbling the turkey until cooked through, about 5 minutes. Taste and adjust seasoning to your liking.

2 Store extras in an airtight container in the fridge for up to 5 days. To reheat, place in a skillet over medium heat while stirring for 3 minutes or until heated through.

Nutritional Info (per serving)				
Calories	Fat	Protein	Carbs	Fiber
400	23g	43g	3g	0.5g

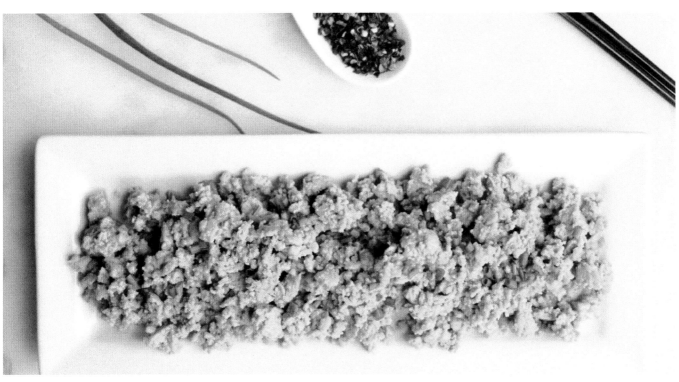

Mexican Shrimp Kabobs

Prep Time: 5 minutes
Cook Time: 6 minutes
Servings: 1

12 medium shrimp, peeled and de-veined
    (I used 2 packages of Sizzlefish shrimp)

2 teaspoons chili powder

1/8 tsp garlic powder

1/8 tsp onion powder

1/8 tsp paprika

1/8 tsp ground cumin

1/4 tsp Celtic sea salt

Avocado oil, for grill

1 Lightly brush grill grates with avocado oil. Preheat grill to medium-high heat. Place 4 wooden skewers in water for 10 minutes.

2 Place the spices in a small bowl and stir well to combine. Liberally sprinkle shrimp with spice mixture. Thread 3 to 4 shrimp onto each skewer. Grill for 3-4 minutes per side or until shrimp is pink and cooked through. Remove from grill and serve. Best served fresh. Can be served cold.

Nutritional Info (per serving)				
Calories	Fat	Protein	Carbs	Fiber
160	1g	35g	4g	2g

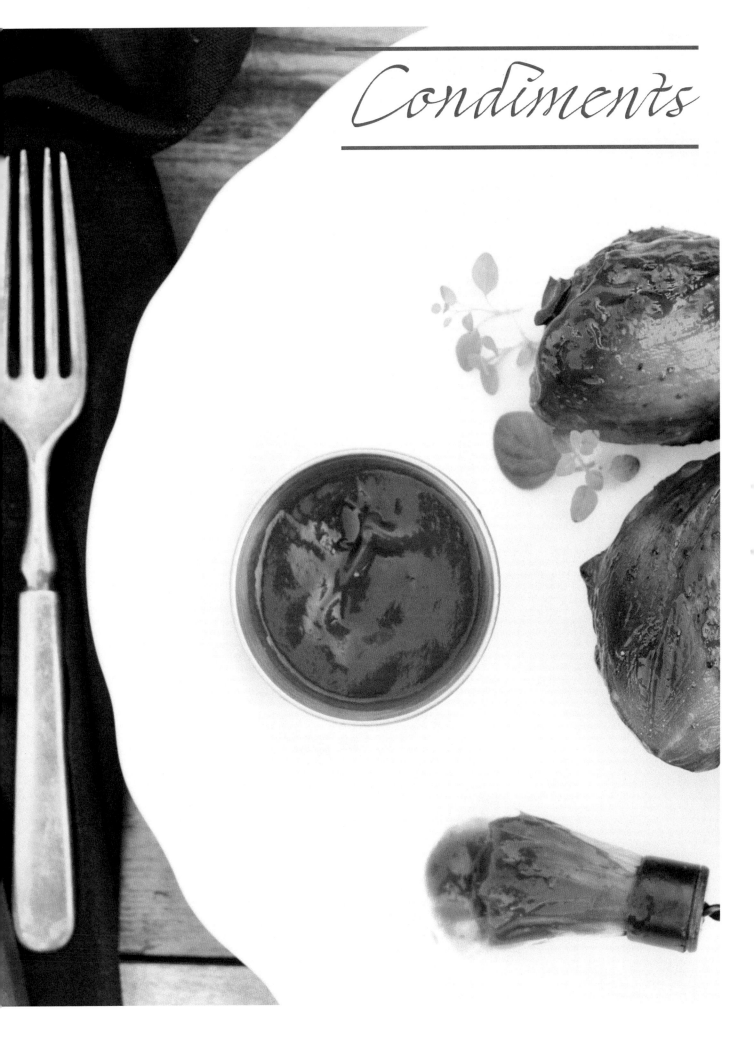

Condiments

Carolina BBQ Sauce

NUT FREE **DAIRY FREE**

Prep Time: 5 minutes
Cook Time: 0 minutes
Servings: 8

1 cup yellow mustard

1 tsp stevia glycerite (or a few drops liquid stevia)

¾ cup coconut vinegar or cider vinegar

1 TBS chili powder

1 tsp ground black pepper

1 tsp ground white pepper

¼ tsp cayenne pepper

2 TBS butter flavored coconut oil, melted

1 tsp liquid smoke

1 Place all the ingredients in a bowl and combine with a spoon until smooth and well mixed (or place into a blender and puree until smooth). Place into an airtight container and store in the fridge for up to 6 days.

Nutritional Info (per serving)				
Calories	Fat	Protein	Carbs	Fiber
36	3g	0.4g	2g	1g

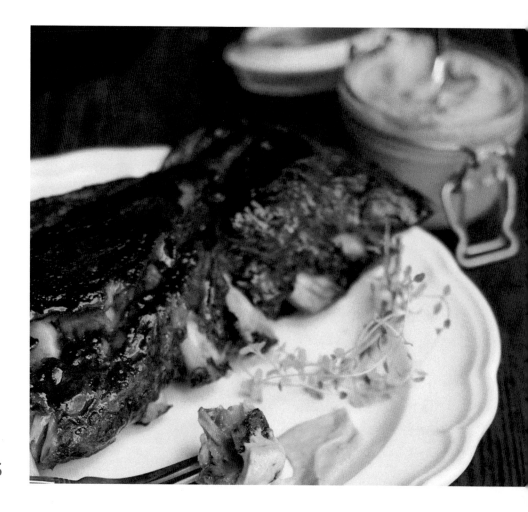

Dijon Vinaigrette

Prep Time: 5 minutes
Cook Time: 0 minutes
Servings: 4

2 tablespoon fresh lemon juice

2 tablespoon Dijon mustard

2 tablespoon apple cider vinegar

1 garlic clove, finely chopped

Sea salt and freshly ground black pepper

1   Whisk lemon juice, Dijon mustard, vinegar, and garlic in a medium bowl. Season with salt and pepper to taste. Use on Pork Chops or store in airtight container in the fridge for up to 6 days.

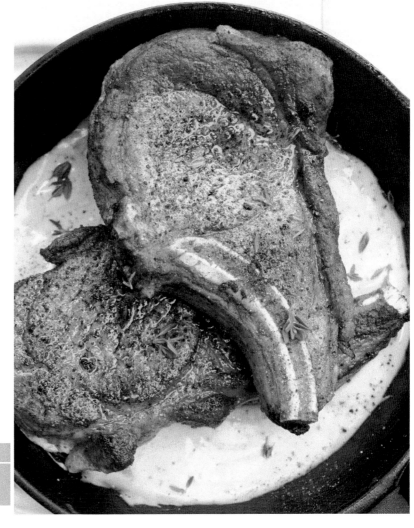

Nutritional Info (per serving)				
Calories	Fat	Protein	Carbs	Fiber
10	0g	0.1g	1g	0.1g

Cilantro Lime Sauce

Prep Time: 5 minutes
Cook Time: 0 minutes
Servings: 4 (1/4 cup per)

¼ cup chicken bone broth (Kettle and Fire brand preferred)

¼ cup fresh cilantro leaves

¼ cup lime juice

1 teaspoon minced garlic

1 teaspoon fine grain sea salt

½ teaspoon ground cumin

½ to 1 small jalapeño pepper (adjust for desired heat), seeded

1 Place all the ingredients in a food processor and puree until smooth.

2 Store in a covered jar in the fridge for up to 8 days.

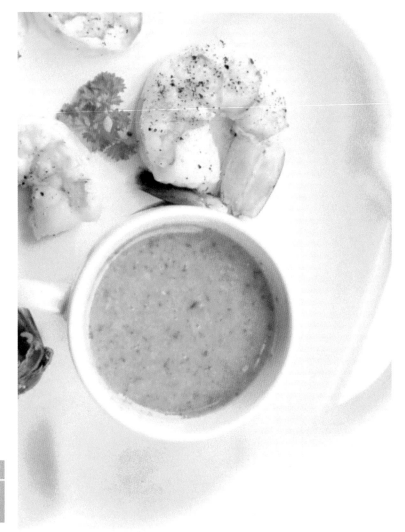

Nutritional Info (per serving)				
Calories	Fat	Protein	Carbs	Fiber
9	0.1g	1g	2g	0.2g

Keto BBQ Sauce

Prep Time: 5 minutes
Cook Time: 0 minutes
Servings: 5 (1/4 cup each)

1 cup tomato sauce

2 tablespoons coconut or apple cider
    vinegar

½ teaspoon onion powder

½ teaspoons garlic powder

Pinch of fine sea salt

½ teaspoons fresh ground pepper

1 teaspoon stevia glycerite or a few drops
    liquid stevia

1½ teaspoons liquid smoke

1   To make the BBQ sauce, place all the ingredients in a large bowl
    and stir well to combine. Taste and adjust sweetness to your
    liking. Store any leftover sauce in an airtight container in the
    refrigerator for up to 8 days.

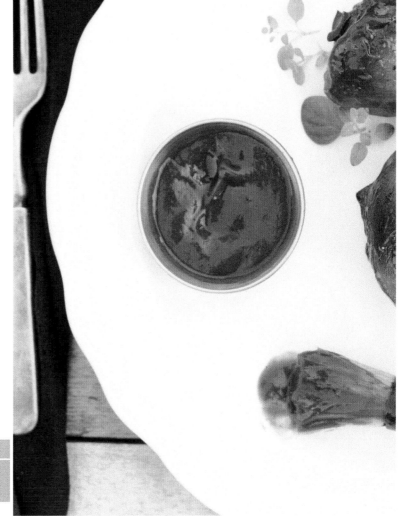

Nutritional Info (per serving)				
Calories	Fat	Protein	Carbs	Fiber
15	0.4g	0.5g	3g	0.5g

Tartar Sauce

Prep Time: 3 minutes
Cook Time: 0 minutes
Servings: 8

½ cup mayo

2 tablespoons dill pickle juice

2 tablespoons dill pickles, diced

1   Combine all ingredients well and serve.

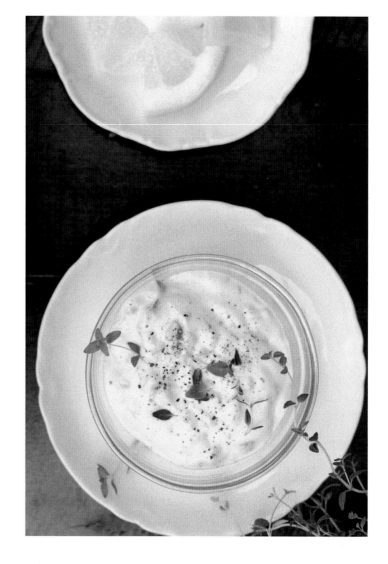

Nutritional Info (per serving)				
Calories	Fat	Protein	Carbs	Fiber
180	20g	0g	0g	0g

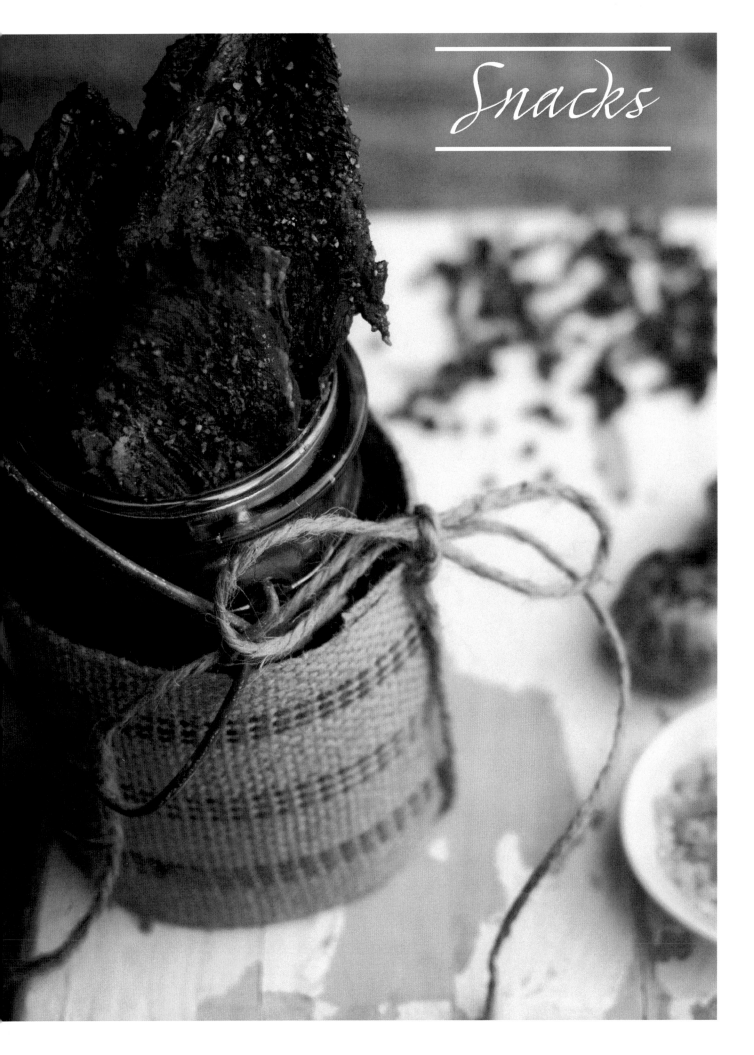

Snacks

Keto (Venison) jerky

NUT FREE **DAIRY FREE**

Prep Time: 5 minutes
Cook Time: 6-8 hours
Servings: 8

1 pound boneless venison or beef loin

MARINADE:

½ cup organic wheat-free tamari

1 tablespoon MCT oil or macadamia nut oil

¼ teaspoon liquid stevia

2 tablespoons lime juice

1 tablespoon grated fresh ginger

1 teaspoon minced garlic

1 teaspoon fine sea salt

1. Place the meat in the freezer for 1 hour to make it easier to slice cleanly. Slice the meat across the grain into long strips, 1 inch wide and ⅛ inch thick.

2. Combine the marinade ingredients in a large shallow bowl. Submerge the strips of meat in the marinade, cover, and marinate in the fridge for at least 2 hours or overnight. Remove the meat from the marinade and sprinkle with the salt.

3. Dehydrator method: Place the strips of meat in a dehydrator, not touching each other, and set the dehydrator to low (170°F).

4. Oven method: If you do not have a dehydrator, preheat the oven to 160°F. Place a rimmed baking sheet on the bottom of the oven (or bottom rack) to catch drips. Arrange the strips of marinated meat directly on the middle rack, not touching each other. Alternatively, place a wire rack on a rimmed baking sheet and arrange the strips of meat on the wire rack.

5. For both methods: Dehydrate the meat for 6 to 8 hours, until the jerky dries to the desired chewiness. For a chewier jerky, dehydrate for less time.

6. Store in an airtight container in the refrigerator for up to 2 weeks or in the freezer for up to a month.

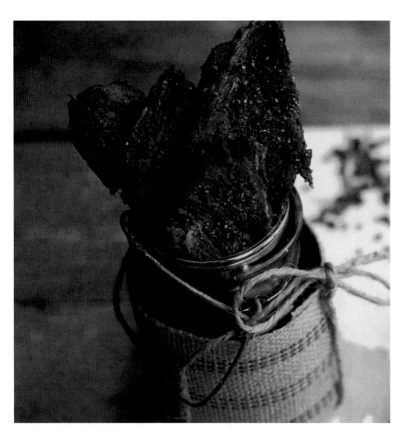

Jerky tastes great and is the ultimate portable food. We often pack it on camping trips. But it is hard to find store-bought jerky that doesn't contain gluten or soy. Thankfully, making homemade jerky is extremely easy; it just takes time to dehydrate. My tip for you is to make a double batch and store it in the freezer.

Nutritional Info (per serving)				
Calories	Fat	Protein	Carbs	Fiber
114	3g	19g	2g	0g

Smoked Jerky

NUT FREE   DAIRY FREE

Prep Time: 10 minutes
Cook Time: 2-3 hours
Servings: 8

1 pound boneless venison or beef loin

MARINADE:

½ cup organic wheat-free tamari

1 tablespoon MCT oil or macadamia nut oil

¼ teaspoon liquid stevia

2 tablespoons lime juice

1 tablespoon grated fresh ginger

1 teaspoon minced garlic

1 teaspoon fine sea salt

Nutritional Info (per serving)				
Calories	Fat	Protein	Carbs	Fiber
114	3g	19g	2g	0g

1. Place the meat in the freezer for 1 hour to make it easier to slice cleanly. Slice the meat across the grain into long strips, 1 inch wide and ⅛ inch thick.

2. Combine the marinade ingredients in a large shallow bowl. Submerge the strips of meat in the marinade, cover, and marinate in the fridge for at least 2 hours or overnight. Remove the meat from the marinade and sprinkle with the salt.

3. Prepare the smoker on low heat adn oil the grate.

4. Lay meat strips on grill so they don't overlap. Smoke over low heat for 2-3 hours or until dried with a hint of moisture in the middle.

5. Store in an airtight container in the refrigerator for up to 2 weeks or in the freezer for up to a month.

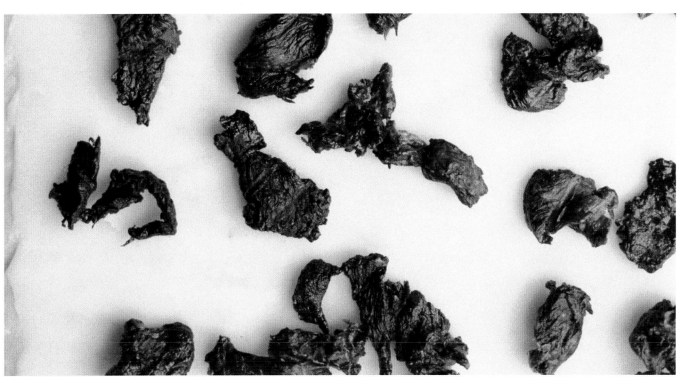

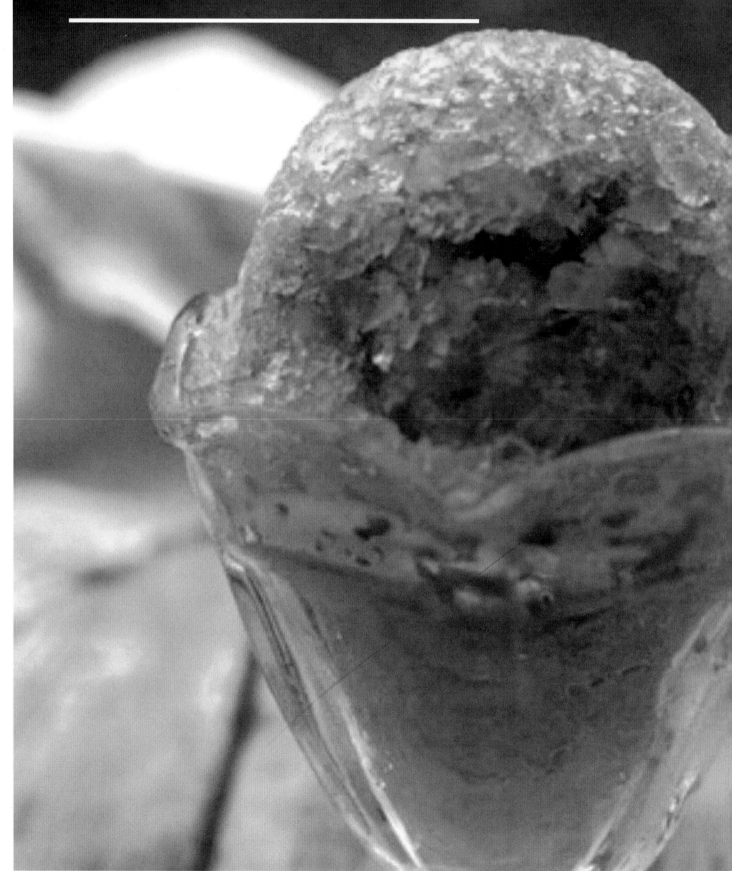

Sweet Treats

Snow Cones

Prep Time: 2 minutes
Cook Time: 0 minutes
Servings: 1

1 cup shaved ice

1 tablespoon Everly mix (any flavor)

2 tablespoons water

1 Shave ice and place into a cup. Mix the Everly into the water. Drizzle over ice and enjoy!

Nutritional Info (per serving)				
Calories	Fat	Protein	Carbs	Fiber
0	0g	0g	0g	0g

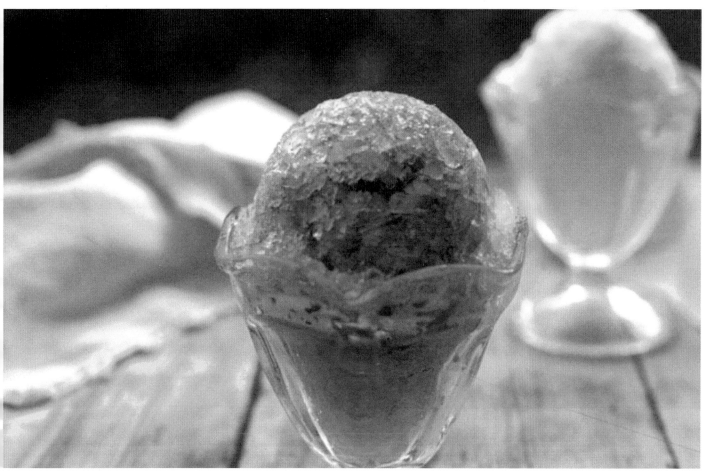

Fruity Ice Popsicles

Prep Time: 5 minutes
Cook Time: 0 minutes
Servings: 4

1 cup water or fizzy water (I used Coconut LaCroix)

1/2 tablespoon Everly drink mix (any flavor)

1/4 teaspoon strawberry stevia (or other fruit flavored stevia such as coconut)

1   Place all ingredients into a blender and purée until well combined. Pour into popsicle mold and place in freezer until totally frozen, about 4 hours. Store in freezer for up to a month.

Nutritional Info (per serving)				
Calories	Fat	Protein	Carbs	Fiber
0	0g	0g	0g	0g

Strawberry Protein Popsicle

Prep Time: 5 minutes
Cook Time: 0 minutes
Servings: 4

1 cup unsweetened almond milk (or unsweetened Hemp milk if nut free)

¼ cup vanilla beef protein powder or egg white protein powder (check for ZERO carbs)

1 teaspoon Strawberry extract

Few drops strawberry stevia

1   Place everything into a blender and puree until smooth. Taste and adjust sweetness to your liking. Pour into popsicle molds and freeze until frozen. Store in freezer for up to a month.

Nutritional Info (per serving)				
Calories	Fat	Protein	Carbs	Fiber
29	1g	5g	0.3g	0.1g

Zero Calorie Slushy

Prep Time: 4 minutes
Cook Time: 0 minutes
Servings: 1

1 cup crushed ice

1 cup water or fizzy water (I used Coconut LaCroix)

1/2 tablespoon Everly drink mix (any flavor)

1/4 teaspoon strawberry stevia (or other fruit flavored stevia such as coconut)

1 Place all ingredients into a blender and purée until smooth. Best served fresh.

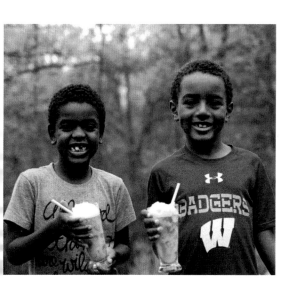

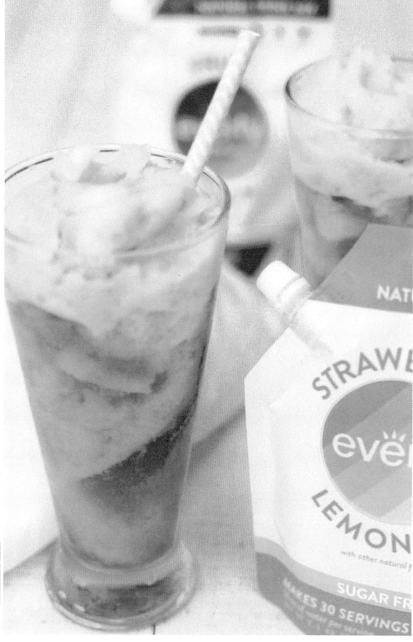

Nutritional Info (per serving)				
Calories	Fat	Protein	Carbs	Fiber
0	0g	0g	0g	0g

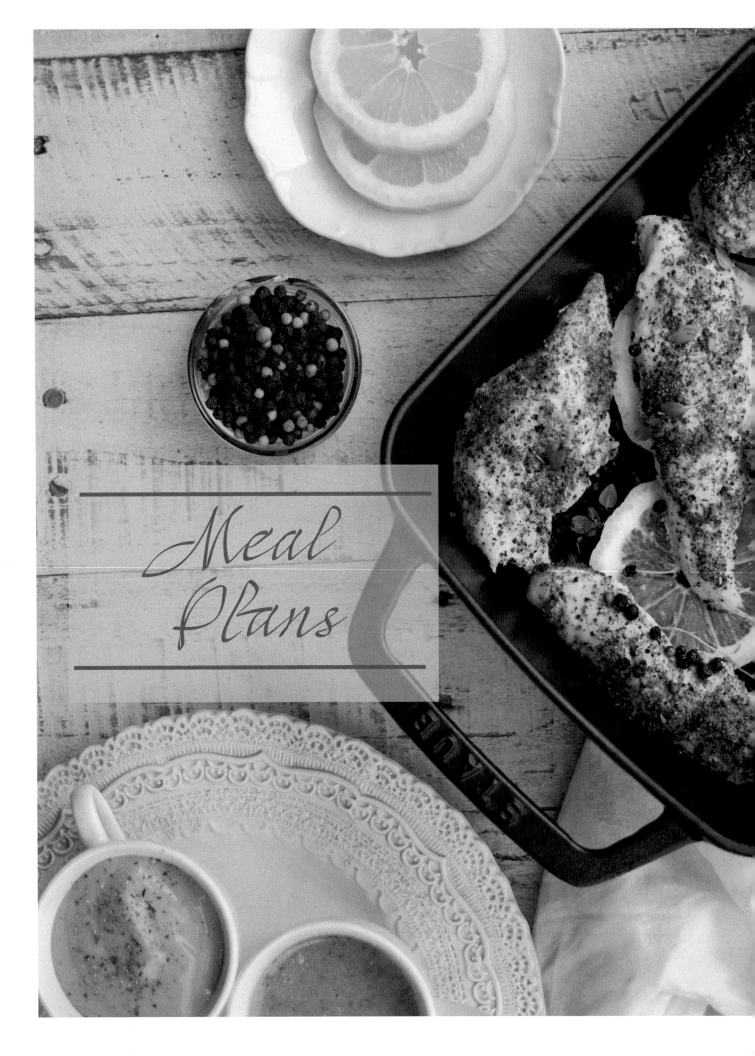

Meal
Plans

Meal Plan Week 1

	Day 1	Day 2	Day 3	Day 4

Day 1

Begin Eating Window

French Toast Porridge

Servings:

Nutritional Info (per serving)

calories	fat	protein	carbs	fiber
195	7g	29g	2g	0.4g

Snack/Side or Dessert

Snow Cones

Servings:

Nutritional Info (per serving)

calories	fat	protein	carbs	fiber
0	0g	0g	0g	0g

End Eating Window

Salt Crusted Fish

Servings:

Nutritional Info (per serving)

calories	fat	protein	carbs	fiber
494	19g	75g	2g	1g

Day 1 Totals

calories	fat	protein	carbs	fiber
689	26g	104g	4g	1.4g

Day 2

Begin Eating Window

Chicken Breakfast Patties

Servings:

Nutritional Info (per serving)

calories	fat	protein	carbs	fiber
289	16g	31g	3g	1g

Snack/Side or Dessert

Keto Venison Jerky

Servings:

Nutritional Info (per serving)

calories	fat	protein	carbs	fiber
114	3g	19g	2g	0g

End Eating Window

Salt Crusted Fish (leftover)

Servings:

Nutritional Info (per serving)

calories	fat	protein	carbs	fiber
494	19g	75g	2g	1g

Day 2 Totals

calories	fat	protein	carbs	fiber
897	38g	125g	7g	2g

Day 3

Begin Eating Window

Ham & Egg White Omelet

Servings:

Nutritional Info (per serving)

calories	fat	protein	carbs	fiber
245	14g	27g	1g	0.1g

Snack/Side or Dessert

Chicken Soup

Servings:

Nutritional Info (per serving)

calories	fat	protein	carbs	fiber
386	15g	58g	2g	0.3g

End Eating Window

Broiled Shrimp with Cilantro Vinaigrette

Servings:

Nutritional Info (per serving)

calories	fat	protein	carbs	fiber
274	14g	35g	4g	0.4g

Day 3 Totals

calories	fat	protein	carbs	fiber
905	43g	120g	7g	0.8g

Day 4

Begin Eating Window

Chicken Breakfast Patties (leftover)

Servings:

Nutritional Info (per serving)

calories	fat	protein	carbs	fiber
289	16g	31g	3g	1g

Snack/Side or Dessert

Keto Venison Jerky (leftover)

Servings:

Nutritional Info (per serving)

calories	fat	protein	carbs	fiber
114	3g	19g	2g	0g

End Eating Window

Keto Fried Rice with Ground Pork

Servings:

Nutritional Info (per serving)

calories	fat	protein	carbs	fiber
341	17g	42g	2g	0.2g

Day 4 Totals

calories	fat	protein	carbs	fiber
744	36g	92g	7g	1.2g

For an interactive version of this meal plan.
http://keto-adapted.com/protein-sparing-modified-fast-ebook-meal-plans/

Meal Plan Week 1 cont.

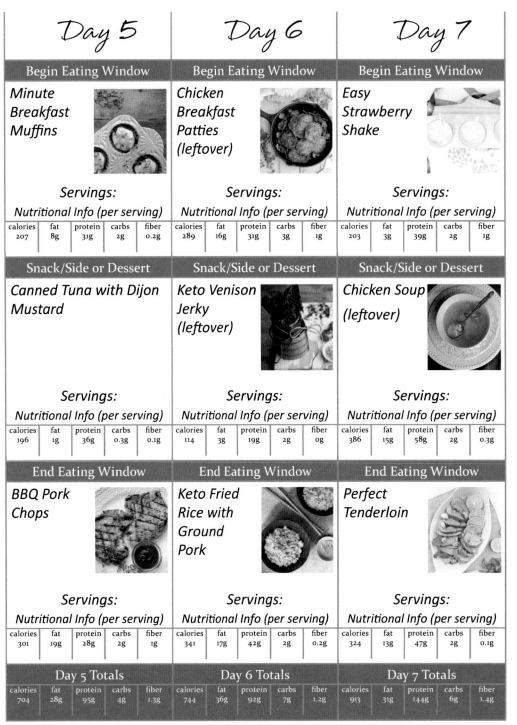

	Day 5	Day 6	Day 7

Day 5

Begin Eating Window

Minute Breakfast Muffins

Servings:
Nutritional Info (per serving)

calories	fat	protein	carbs	fiber
207	8g	31g	2g	0.2g

Snack/Side or Dessert

Canned Tuna with Dijon Mustard

Servings:
Nutritional Info (per serving)

calories	fat	protein	carbs	fiber
196	1g	36g	0.3g	0.1g

End Eating Window

BBQ Pork Chops

Servings:
Nutritional Info (per serving)

calories	fat	protein	carbs	fiber
301	19g	28g	2g	1g

Day 5 Totals

calories	fat	protein	carbs	fiber
704	28g	95g	4g	1.3g

Day 6

Begin Eating Window

Chicken Breakfast Patties (leftover)

Servings:
Nutritional Info (per serving)

calories	fat	protein	carbs	fiber
289	16g	31g	3g	1g

Snack/Side or Dessert

Keto Venison Jerky (leftover)

Servings:
Nutritional Info (per serving)

calories	fat	protein	carbs	fiber
114	3g	19g	2g	0g

End Eating Window

Keto Fried Rice with Ground Pork

Servings:
Nutritional Info (per serving)

calories	fat	protein	carbs	fiber
341	17g	42g	2g	0.2g

Day 6 Totals

calories	fat	protein	carbs	fiber
744	36g	92g	7g	1.2g

Day 7

Begin Eating Window

Easy Strawberry Shake

Servings:
Nutritional Info (per serving)

calories	fat	protein	carbs	fiber
203	3g	39g	2g	1g

Snack/Side or Dessert

Chicken Soup (leftover)

Servings:
Nutritional Info (per serving)

calories	fat	protein	carbs	fiber
386	15g	58g	2g	0.3g

End Eating Window

Perfect Tenderloin

Servings:
Nutritional Info (per serving)

calories	fat	protein	carbs	fiber
324	13g	47g	2g	0.1g

Day 7 Totals

calories	fat	protein	carbs	fiber
913	31g	144g	6g	1.4g

Note:

This meal plan will have extra servings at the end of the week. So you can either repeat until leftovers are done or freeze them for another week.

On Keto-Adapted.com you can adjust serving sizes as needed.

Grocery List Week 1

Baking Products

Beef bone broth	1/2 cups
Chicken bone broth	8 cups
Lime juice	3 tablespoons

Canned Items

Canned tuna (two 5-ounce cans)	10 ounces
Capers	2 tablespoons

Condiments

Dijon mustard	1/4 cups
Organic Tamari	1/2 cups

Eggs

Egg whites	28 large
Eggs	12 large

Fats and Oils

Coconut oil	1/4 cups
Lard (or more coconut oil)	1 teaspoon
MCT oil	1 tablespoons

Fresh Herbs

Fresh chives	2 tablespoons
Fresh dill	2 tablespoons
Fresh ginger	1 tablespoons
Fresh thyme (or parsley)	0.12 cups

Milk and Drinks

Unsweetened almond milk	1.67 cups
Everly Mix (any flavor)	1 tablespoons

Produce

Garlic	5 cloves
Lemon	1
Onion	1/2 cup
Scallions	1

Protein Powder

Unflavored egg white protein powder	1/2 cup

Proteins

Bone-in pork loin chops	20 ounces
Chicken breasts	3 large
Ground chicken	16 ounces
Ground chicken	48 ounces
Ham sliced (4 inch diameter)	6 slices
Ham (chopped or cubed)	2 ounces
Shrimp	8 ounces
Trout	48 ounces
Venison tenderloin	16 ounces

Spices and Extracts

Celery salt	1/2 teaspoon
Crushed red pepper flakes	1 teaspoon
Dried thyme	2 teaspoons
Fine grain sea salt	7 teaspoons
Fresh ground black pepper	2 teaspoon
Ground cinnamon	1 sprinkle
Ground nutmeg	1/2 teaspoon
Maple extract	1/2 teaspoon
Paprika	1 teaspoon
Sage (dried and ground)	1 tablespoon
Sea salt	2 cups
Strawberry extract	1 teaspoon

Sweeteners

Confectioners Swerve	1/4 cups
Stevia glycerite	1/2 teaspoon
Strawberry stevia	1 drop

Meal Plan Week 2

	Day 1	Day 2	Day 3	Day 4

Begin Eating Window

	Day 1	Day 2	Day 3	Day 4
Meal	French Toast Porridge	Easy Strawberry Shake	Ham & Egg White Omelet	Minute Breakfast Muffins
Servings:				

	calories	fat	protein	carbs	fiber
Day 1	195	7g	29g	2g	0.4g
Day 2	203	3g	39g	2g	1g
Day 3	245	14g	27g	1g	0.1g
Day 4	207	8g	31g	2g	0.2g

Snack/Side or Dessert

	Day 1	Day 2	Day 3	Day 4
Meal	Shrimp Fried Rice	Keto Bread Sandwich	Shrimp Fried Rice (leftover)	Keto Bread Sandwich (leftover)
Servings:		Eat 2 servings		Eat 2 servings

	calories	fat	protein	carbs	fiber
Day 1	183	5g	32g	2g	0.2g
Day 2	64	0.2g	14g	0.8g	0g
Day 3	183	5g	32g	2g	0.2g
Day 4	64	0.2g	14g	0.4g	0g

End Eating Window

	Day 1	Day 2	Day 3	Day 4
Meal	Lean Hamburger Patties with Mustard	Grilled Chicken Breasts with Carolina BBQ	Simple Poached Turkey Breast	Grilled Chicken Breasts with Carolina BBQ (leftover)
Servings:				

	calories	fat	protein	carbs	fiber
Day 1	312	11g	49g	1g	0.4g
Day 2	304	13g	43g	2g	1g
Day 3	257	4g	52g	0.1g	0g
Day 4	304	13g	43g	2g	1g

Day Totals

	calories	fat	protein	carbs	fiber
Day 1 Totals	690	23g	110g	5g	1g
Day 2 Totals	571	16g	96g	4g	2g
Day 3 Totals	685	23g	111g	3g	0.5g
Day 4 Totals	571	21g	88g	4g	1.2g

Meal Plan Week 2 cont.

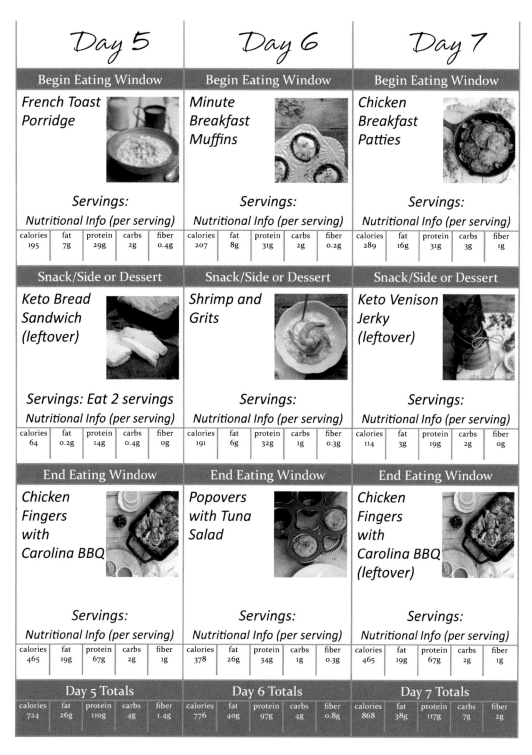

	Day 5					Day 6					Day 7			
Begin Eating Window					**Begin Eating Window**					**Begin Eating Window**				
French Toast Porridge					Minute Breakfast Muffins					Chicken Breakfast Patties				
Servings:					Servings:					Servings:				

Nutritional Info (per serving)

calories	fat	protein	carbs	fiber		calories	fat	protein	carbs	fiber		calories	fat	protein	carbs	fiber
195	7g	29g	2g	0.4g		207	8g	31g	2g	0.2g		289	16g	31g	3g	1g

Snack/Side or Dessert

Day 5: Keto Bread Sandwich (leftover) — Servings: Eat 2 servings

Day 6: Shrimp and Grits — Servings:

Day 7: Keto Venison Jerky (leftover) — Servings:

Nutritional Info (per serving)

calories	fat	protein	carbs	fiber		calories	fat	protein	carbs	fiber		calories	fat	protein	carbs	fiber
64	0.2g	14g	0.4g	0g		191	6g	32g	1g	0.3g		114	3g	19g	2g	0g

End Eating Window

Day 5: Chicken Fingers with Carolina BBQ — Servings:

Day 6: Popovers with Tuna Salad — Servings:

Day 7: Chicken Fingers with Carolina BBQ (leftover) — Servings:

Nutritional Info (per serving)

calories	fat	protein	carbs	fiber		calories	fat	protein	carbs	fiber		calories	fat	protein	carbs	fiber
465	19g	67g	2g	1g		378	26g	34g	1g	0.3g		465	19g	67g	2g	1g

Day 5 Totals					Day 6 Totals					Day 7 Totals				
calories	fat	protein	carbs	fiber	calories	fat	protein	carbs	fiber	calories	fat	protein	carbs	fiber
724	26g	110g	4g	1.4g	776	40g	97g	4g	0.8g	868	38g	117g	7g	2g

Note:

This meal plan will have extra servings at the end of the week. So you can either repeat until leftovers are done or freeze them for another week.

On Keto-Adapted.com you can adjust serving sizes as needed.

Grocery List Week 2

Baking Products

Aluminum free baking powder	1 teaspoon
Beef bone broth	1/2 cups

Canned Items

Canned tuna (two 5-ounce cans)	10 ounces

Condiments

Dijon mustard	1/4 cup
Mayonnaise	2 tablespoons
Mustard	3/4 cup
Organic Tamari	2 teaspoons

Eggs

Egg whites	70 large
(about 3 1/2 32-ounce boxes of all whites)	
Eggs	4 large

Fats and Oils

Coconut oil	6 tablespoons

Fresh Herbs

Fresh chives	1/4 cups
Fresh flat-leaf parsley (for garnish)	

Milk and Drinks

Unsweetened almond milk	5 1/3 cups

Produce

Garlic	2 clove
Lemon	1
Onion (chopped)	1/4 cups
Scallions	1

Protein Powder

Unflavored egg white protein powder	1 1/4 cups

Proteins

Bacon	3 strips
Chicken breasts (2 pounds)	8 large
Ground beef 95% lean	16 ounces
Ground chicken (or turkey)	48 ounces
Ham	24 slices
Ham sliced (4 inch diameter)	12 slices
Ham (chopped or cubed)	2 ounces
Shrimp (peeled and deveined)	16 ounces
Shrimp	12 large
Turkey breast (one 3-pound)	48 ounces

Spices and Extracts

Celery salt (or regular salt)	1/2 teaspoon
Crushed red pepper flakes	2 teaspoons
Dried thyme (chopped)	2 teaspoons
Fine grain sea salt	1/4 cup
Fresh ground black pepper	5 teaspoons
Garlic powder	1/2 teaspoon
Ground cinnamon	2 sprinkle
Ground nutmeg	1/2 teaspoon
Italian seasoning	1 teaspoon
Lemon pepper seasoning	2 tablespoons
Maple extract	3 tablespoons
Paprika	1 teaspoon
Sage (dried and ground)	1 tablespoon
Strawberry extract	1 teaspoon

Sweeteners

Confectioners Swerve	1/2 cups
Stevia glycerite	1/2 teaspoon
Strawberry stevia	1 drop

For an interactive version of this meal plan.
http://keto-adapted.com/protein-sparing-modified-fast-ebook-meal-plan

Keto-Adapted.com

Click Here to see all the features of our subscription site keto-adapted.com.

Some of the features you get are:

- Exclusive educational and tutorial videos

- Articles on the latest Science

- Live Weekly Webinars with Craig and Maria

- Interactive Meal Planner to drag and drop recipes and automatically calculate daily macros

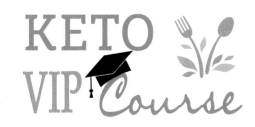

Go Here to get started: Keto-Adapted.com

NEW Courses!

Brand new Keto Courses are the best way to start your keto journey or to learn even more about how this can be a lifestyle for your whole family. Just some of what is included:

- Weekly Live webinars with Maria and Craig

- Lifetime access including new content each year

- Over 75 amazing videos and cooking instruction

- Handouts and downloadable documents to help keep you on track

- Up to 90 day of interactive online meal plans!

Go Here to get started: Keto-Adapted.com/School

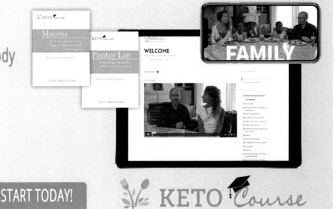

THE KETO COURSE
Everything you need to Lose Weight and Heal your Body

- Lifetime Access
- 8 weekly Live webinars
- Over 75 amazing videos (with closed captions)
- Up to 60 days of Interactive Meal Plans
- How to get your whole Family keto!
- Eating keto at restaurants
- Exclusive member access and much more!

START TODAY!

KETO Course

65 - Meal Plans

Made in the USA
Las Vegas, NV
18 January 2022

41645625R00040